W9-CFM-046

Runner's World
STRETCHING BOOK

Runner's World
STRETCHING BOOK

by Nell Weaver

Runner's World Books

Library of Congress Cataloging in Publication Data

Weaver, Nell.

Runner's World Stretching Book.

(Instructional book series; 12)

Bibliography: p.

1 Running- -Training 2. Exercise. 3. Muscle strength. 4. Stretch
(Physiology) I. Runner's world. II. Title. III: Stretching book.

GV1061.5.W4 1982   613.7'1   82-12372

ISBN 0-89037-242-X

ISBN 0-89037-234-9 (pbk.)

Runner's World Books

in conjunction with

Anderson World, Inc., Mountain View, California

Contents

Dedication

To Bob, my favorite running partner

Acknowledgments

I would like to extend my appreciation to:

B.K.S. Iyengar, of Poona, India, the yoga teacher whose experiential work with the human body has greatly influenced my views on physical and mental conditioning; Janet Downs, of Cambridge, England, my first Iyengar-style teacher, whose creative, disciplined approach to realizing a healthy body continues to challenge my own efforts; Jean Couch, my friend, and co-author of *Runner's World Yoga Book*; Ellen Simpson and Gary Harper, M.D., for their editorial comments; Marian Garfinkel, of Philadelphia, Judith Lasater and Ramanand Patel of San Francisco's Institute for Yoga Teacher Education, Kathy Richardson, the Sparkling River Farm, Lone Thorstensen of Denmark, and George F. Weaver, the teachers and friends who have influenced my views on exercise and life; my students, some of whom have been working and stretching with me for many years; my mother, Hannah Weaver, an excellent recreational walker, and my dad, George D. Weaver, who serves as her coach.

I would like to thank Don Peccerill for appearing with me in the stretching photos. Photography is by David Keith.

Introduction

A running friend of mine once told me that although he stretched regularly, he was still plagued with miserably tight legs and a stiff, aching back. He confessed that he was considering giving up either stretching or his running, or perhaps even both.

"Show me how you stretch," I asked him.

"Oh, you know, I just do all those stretches you're supposed to do."

"Like what? C'mon, let's see your typical stretching workout."

"Well, let's see. I do a little of this."

He took his legs about five feet apart, bent over and bounced quickly up and down. His knees buckled, his face became horribly contorted, but he kept on bouncing.

"And I do a lot of this one."

He stood up, brought his feet closer together, threw his arms out, and twisted stiffly back and forth from the waist. His lips sucked in air and determinedly blew it out. His face got red; he was working hard.

"Sometimes I finish off with this."

He lay down, quickly rolled his hips up off the floor, supported his buttocks with his hands, and let his legs and bent knees hang over his face. His toes strained to touch the floor, bounced there for a few seconds, and then were suspended in the air behind his head. His eyes and lips were clenched. His breath was forced, his neck was turning purple, and he was moaning softly.

I knelt beside his face.

"You look awfully uncomfortable."

Suddenly, his body snapped open like a pocketknife. He was on his back, looking up at me with confused eyes.

"But, Nell, these exercises were in a book!"

Perhaps they were — or perhaps something very much like them exists somewhere in some book. Unfortunately, my friend was not utilizing his body or the exercise action correctly. I worked with him for a few minutes, and showed him how, by using a different body position and different movements, he could achieve benefits from the exercises he had chosen.

That's the goal of any exercise program: positive change. If you don't feel better after exercising, you probably were doing something wrong. This could involve subtleties in your diet, your training schedule, your mental or emotional approach to exercise, your technique or style, your equipment, and so on.

And if you're stretching regularly, and feeling worse instead of better after your stretching session, you're doing something wrong. Hopefully, this book can help.

If stretching is new for you, I'm glad you've discovered the method in this book. Stretching exercises can bring a new dimension to your fitness commitment. If you enjoy working with this book, perhaps you'll want to find a good yoga teacher or dance/ movement coach. But remember, no matter how many great instructors you may have during your life — you control your own fitness level and well-being.

Happy stretching!

Nell Weaver
Little Rock, Arkansas
May, 1982

1

The Running Body

Running has become America's passion. During the last decade it has left the confinements of elite athletics and entered the conversations, over morning coffee, of fifty-year-old housewives. Business has turned its attention to the sport, too: Madison Avenue perceives runners as desirable and loyal consumers; corporate sponsorship of races continues to grow. Sometimes it seems like every man and woman in America is either a runner or married to one.

There are many good reasons behind the popularity of running. It is one of the most efficient means to achieve cardiovascular fitness. Running allows you to maintain a healthy body weight, with a decreased percentage of total body fat. The mental benefits, although of a more subjective nature, have been pointed out by fitness experts and by those who run. The movement of running is relatively simple and perhaps an inherently natural physical action. The sport may be enjoyed almost anywhere, too, and beyond a good pair of shoes, there is no essential equipment. Running can be enjoyed with or without a companion.

But there are a few negative side effects: running can lead to a tight, inflexible lower body and a disproportionately weak upper body. Anyone who concentrates on a specific sport will invariably strengthen certain muscles, but there will also be those opposing muscle groups that are not strengthened. This imbalance is struck because movement occurs when certain muscles contract. Repeated contractions result in a shortened muscle. The muscle spindle—the message center of the muscle—responds by becoming resistant to lengthening. This process determines the length of the muscle at rest. If muscles are allowed to shorten, they can have several effects: inhibit joint movement, deprive their opposing muscle group of optimum development and increase the chance of injury.

The act of running involves contracting the muscles along the back of the leg and buttocks. The opposing muscle groups, in the front of the leg, are relatively weakened. Running also involves a bounding movement that causes the heels to strike the earth and absorb as much as three times the body's weight on each foot strike. This repeated striking action affects the back and spine. Backside muscles tighten, which can reduce mobility in the knee and hip joint. Excessively inflexible hamstrings (the result of running) can affect the back and cause joint misalignment.

Besides the annoying feelings of stiffness that a runner's tight muscles brings, his body may also be ripe for an even more serious occurrence—painful injury. Experience tells us, and research confirms, that anytime one muscle group is overdeveloped, the odds of injury in the opposing weaker muscle group increase dramatically.

The runner also unknowingly experiences microscopic tears in his musculature during long runs. These tears in the fascia—the connective tissue of the body—result in scar tissue. Scar tissue is not readily pliable, but fortunately, inhibited joint mobility, and muscular tightness caused by a buildup of scar tissue, can be counteracted by routine stretching.

Beginning runners encounter yet another problem: overuse injuries. Muscles that have not been stressed in their past sedentary role and that are suddenly put to work will feel the strain. Overuse among novice runners invariably causes problems, according to Little Rock running coach Deb Strehle: "Beginners can demand too much, too fast. The most common injuries I see with my beginning runners involve classic cases of overuse."

Strehle, a former cross-country competitor for the University of Kansas, has completed seventeen marathons. Her experience with running gives her keen insight to overuse injuries. She heartily recommends stretching exercises for her runners; stretching is good protection against overuse injuries and applies to runners of all abilities; however, she finds stretching to be an essential ingredient in a beginning runner's program.

The runner's usually underdeveloped upper body and accompanying leg stretch imbalance can also be improved through alternate exercises and stretching. The exercises in this book emphasize flexibility and strength conditioning. A regular stretching program should be considered good sound preventive work that can enhance your running, no matter how long you have been on the roads. The creation of a fit, flexible running body will happen if you exercise regularly, and if you stretch correctly.

2

What Happens When You Stretch

There are two basic stretching methods: ballistic and static. The ballistic approach is the traditional "up-two-three" philosophy of what exercise should be. Drill sergeants leading exercises for their army recruits would be a good example of the "ballistic mentality." It is usually associated with an attitude of aggressively forcing or pushing the body through pain barriers. Stretching movements are repeated quickly and with a bouncing action. Ironically, ballistic stretching tends to tighten muscles and cause soreness. Also, instead of providing the expected injury-preventive benefits, ballistic stretching itself can be a cause of injury.

Here's why the ballistic stretch is bad. When a muscle is jerked into extension, its message center responds by shortening or tightening the muscle. This quick contraction is a means of self-protection against overstretching. The result is that the muscles supposedly being stretched are actually being tightened!

The "touch your hands ten times to the floor" routine has another danger. Athletes using a quick, bouncing action to stretch may not realize when they have bounced past the body's current stretching limit. This lack of awareness can lead to an injury from stretching.

Static stretching, on the other hand, uses slow, sustained, rhythmic movements. The athlete takes an exercise position designed to stretch specific muscles. The position is held or sustained, while the message center of the muscle being stretched receives a clear signal to lengthen; the muscle becomes less sensitive to being stretched and responds by increasing its resting length.

The static-stretch approach to "ballistic toe touching" is a slow hang. The body is bent at the hips and the arms droop downward. The hamstring muscles of the legs can now lengthen and become more flexible. The slower, rhythmical technique of static stretching also allows for an awareness of stretching limits, something which is absent in ballistic bouncing. As a result, the likelihood of a stretching injury is greatly reduced.

Static stretching has another conditioning benefit. The slow, sustained stretch of one group of muscles involves a sustained contraction of the opposing muscle group. So when athletes focus on stretching muscles, they will also be strengthening muscles (through sustained contraction) that would not otherwise be developed in their sports. For example, distance runners who target the backs of the legs as an area to be stretched will also be able to strengthen the muscles of the front of the legs, which are relatively weakened in running.

3

How to Make
Stretching Work for You

"Everyone I run with respects stretching." These are the words of a veteran woman runner. During her years on the road, Pat Torvestad has shared the miles with a diverse group of runners. She was the first woman from Arkansas to compete in the Boston Marathon. She runs regularly with the celebrated cross-country enthusiasts, Hash House Harriers, and with the lesser-known, but equally colorful, Marquis de Sade Running Club of Little Rock, Arkansas. Their members are dedicated to early morning runs of many miles with many hills. Torvestad also ran on the 1980 Lake Placid Winter Olympic Games torch relay team; during her one-hundred-mile stint with this team, she regularly used stretching exercises for warmups and cooldowns:

"The participants in the best all-around shape" Torvestad said, "were usually better prepared to sustain the pace. We would run in the extreme cold, jump back into the van while someone else ran, dash off to a ceremony, climb back in the van, and then it would be time to crawl out and run again. Stretching whenever possible really helped!"

Gary Smith, the manager of a popular running store in Little Rock, and an accomplished runner himself, says he finds time to stretch while tending the business. Smith says he tries to do stretching exercises during his day in the store, as well as before his runs. He adds that his weekly maintenance level of fifty to sixty miles is less hampered by injury when he is stretching regularly throughout his workday.

Regular stretching can benefit you, just as it has Pat and Gary. And static stretching is such a simple concept. You can break static stretching into three components: (1) moving slowly into the stretching position, (2) holding the position for several breaths or seconds, and (3) slowly releasing the hold. Each part of the process is equally important. Let's take a closer look at each step.

Moving slowly into the stretching position – In order to maximize the effectiveness of the stretch, your body should be properly aligned according to the exercise instructions. Movement into the stretch should be slow in order to maintain this alignment and to reduce the risk of injury. If you move too quickly, your momentum could take your body too far into a stretch. Most major movements in static stretching should be done with quiet, steady exhalations.

Holding the stretch – Once you have positioned your body, hold the stretch. Strength and flexibility differ among individuals, so it's impossible to specify a definite, fixed length of time for the hold. As your flexibility improves, you will be able to hold the stretch longer. But a word of warning. Overstretching is a dangerous temptation for many athletes, and holding a stretch for too long is a form of overstretching. Disturbing or changing the alignment of the body during the stretch can also cause overstretching. Perhaps most importantly, in addition to relaxing the body part being stretched, you should also relax the muscles in your face and neck.

Breathe normally through the nose while stretching. Breath awareness, and its role in stretching movements, may be a foreign concept to you. If so, concentrate on your breathing sometime when you are standing or sitting quietly. Focus only on the breathing. Check both the inhalation and the exhalation for their quality of regularity, length and evenness. While monitoring your breath do not alter it in any way. It may be useful before each stretching session to pause and identify your regular breathing pattern before working with your breath while stretching.

Sometimes you may find a stretch is uncomfortable or painful. Eventually you'll learn how to work through discomfort, but you should never work with pain. Learn to distinguish between discomfort and pain by "listening" to your body. Use your common sense. Pain is like an alarm clock buzzer—a signal meant to be noticed. If you experience pain during a stretch, release the position immediately. Examine the exercise instructions again, if you're following a program. Check for alignment advice and study the illustration. Try to make the stretch less intense by using an easier variation. Since overstretching is an ineffective way to exercise, it may actually be better for you to work with a stretch that doesn't seem too demanding. After a few days, try the more challenging version.

Release the stretch slowly — Focus on your alignment and use the same slow, steady breath that took you into the stretch, as you leave your stretch position. You'll lose the positive stretching and strengthening benefits of the release movement if you leave the stretch too quickly, and you may injure yourself. However, sometimes you will lose control during a stretch, and this will prevent your control of the release movement. Your body is learning a new movement, and so its inability to sustain a smooth, controlled action in the beginning, is inevitable. If you felt awkward coming out of a stretch, try again. It also helps to have a sense of humor in any stretching exercise program.

There are other aspects of stretching that we will consider here. But remember—the most important rule is to stretch!

Q. How often should I stretch?

A. The easy answer is "whenever you can." If you are already involved in a regular sports exercise routine, you will need to make time for your stretching, just as you would schedule any other activity. Regularity is the magic word in any exercise program. The novice stretcher should set aside a ten- to fifteen-minute time slot in the morning or evening. If you're stretching in conjunction with running or another sport, add fifteen minutes to each training session to allow time for warming up and cooling down. Understanding that stretching does take time, and working this time into your daily routine, will help give you "time to stretch."

There will be other more impromptu stretching opportunities every day. For example, examine your body position while waiting in a line, talking on the telephone, watching TV, or preparing a meal. Seize any opportunity for a good stretch.

Q. What type of clothing should I stretch in?

A. Wear anything that is loose, comfortable and allows you to move freely. If you're stretching inside on a smooth floor or outside on grass, for example, you can work with bare feet. You might slip wearing socks or stocking-type tights. Covering the feet during indoor exercise inhibits movement. You need to be able to stretch and easily work the feet.

Q. Where should I stretch?

A. Wherever there's enough room for you to move. Ideally, you'll find a clean, flat space. Carpeted floors are acceptable, but bare floors are better. (Use a blanket or mat when you do exercises that require some padding.) You'll be glad you're on a bare floor when you're performing standing exercises in which sure footing is essential.

If you're stretching outside, try to do it on grass, so you can remove your shoes and socks. Sometimes grass is not available or appropriate to your outdoor setting, but at least choose a spot that is smooth and level. If you're stretching outside in the summer months, do it in the shade.

Q. Which exercises are most important?

A. When starting, use the exercise guides in Chapter 9, or simply choose exercises to fit the needs of your stretching session (i.e., warmups or cooldowns). Learn to "listen" to your body so that you can find stretches to counteract its weak areas. When you do exercises that are repeated on either side of the body, you may discover you like exercises on one side, and ones that are perhaps more difficult on the other side and, therefore, not as pleasing. But try to balance the length of your stretching regimen by incorporating both types into your exercise schedule. A stretching position that is difficult indicates you're probably working an inflexible area that really needs to be stretched.

Q. How long should I hold a stretch?

A. The duration of the stretching position will depend on your present state of flexibility and strength. Your stretching capacity will change daily; it will even vary from hour to hour. Certainly it will improve with regular stretching. Your stretching capacity will not be greatly benefited, however, by competition. So use the illustrations as guides, but don't compete with them. In fact, competition serves no useful purpose in stretching, so ignore the flexibility capabilities of your companions. Work within the framework of your own body. Listen to it, challenge it, but never abuse it by forcing it into a competitive position. When competition is used in a stretch, self-awareness is absent.

The length of time indicated for holding a stretch is a suggestion; adjust the time to meet your own needs. Remember that you can work effectively with discomfort, but not with pain.

Q. What about my breathing?

A. Your breathing should be natural, and not forced, loud or intense. Breathe quietly through your nose. Never hold your breath during an exercise. At first, take a "breath check" periodically to make sure you're not holding your breath, breathing through your mouth, or breathing noisily. Most of the major movements in this book should be done with slow, steady exhalations. You may find yourself spontaneously initiating a deeper, longer breath during a stretch, or you may breathe more quickly, and your breath may seem to originate higher in the chest. If a breathing pattern change does occur spontaneously, see if it aids you in the stretch.

The successful augmentation of the breath in stretching is basically a test of your ability to observe these unsolicited changes, plus your willingness to cooperate with your breathing. Work with your breath and not against it. Never force the breath. This only creates unnecessary tension.

Q. Can stretching aid my relaxation?

A. Relaxation through stretching can happen if you utilize the correct stretching techniques....and if you forget your gym class training. Forget jerking from side to side or bouncing up and down like a yo-yo. Eliminate the athletic foundation of goals and objectives. Save your training schedule and records for your sport.

Refuse to be bound by the notion of what your body "can and can't do." Rejoice instead in your own movement and experience fully your own interpretations of the stretching exercises. Elongate your spine and limbs and create more space within your body. Keep an open, receptive attitude during each stretching session.

Any unnecessary effort (for example, creating an artificial breathing pattern) is a waste of muscular tension and energy. Obviously you must work the muscles that are necessary to hold the stretch, but you'll never need to carry tension in your face or neck. Also, watch for and avoid unnecessary tightness in the shoulders or abdomen. During your stretches, take note from day to day of places you find yourself routinely tightening or contracting. If you are involved in sports, perhaps those tension spots are also present during your workouts. An awareness of a muscle tightening where it is not necessary, and its subsequent elimination, can lead to a more relaxed and more efficient athletic movement.

You may also discover these same tension areas at other times during the day. This extra tension saps energy and can also take the form of a headache, neck or back pain, and so on. That's why stretching is a routine to consider using at all hours of the day or night. Emulate your dog or cat; they intersperse stretching throughout the day.

Q. Can I stretch with an injury?

A. Avoiding use of the injured tissue is probably the best therapy. This might mean an extended layoff from your athletic activity, or you may be able to continue stretching, as long as it doesn't involve the injured area. Monitor your body and use your common sense. Consult a sports physician or a physical therapist if you're unsure of the recommended treatment.

Q. Can stretching help eliminate lower-back pain?

A. Many of the stretches in this book are very good for preventing or relieving back pain. Key on the exercises designed to correctly align the pelvic area. Some exercises teach you to bend with a "flat back." This is just another way to emulate the movement of a concave spine that bends primarily at the hips, instead of at the waist, or by rounding the shoulders. However, if you have a weak back, you may want to avoid this position when starting out, or use a more gentle back action, as in the Roll Down Hang. If back pain drastically prohibits your movement, try some of the resting positions found at the end of Cooldowns, Chapter 8.

Q. Can I stretch if I have special physical concerns?

A. The maximum utilization of exercise is up to you. This is true even if you have special physical limitations. If you are unsure about using the exercises in this book, show them to your doctor or therapist for his recommendation. Adjust the exercise positions to fit your own ability and needs. Remember that stretching exercises are not competitive, so try to let go of any frustrations you may feel while stretching. Approach stretching positively and work *with* your body.

Q. Can the elderly stretch?

A. Stretching may be safely begun at any age. If you are already physically active, the exercises in this book can enhance your sports enjoyment. If exercise is a new activity for you, then stretching may become a fantastic route to improving muscle tone and making joints more limber. Whether active or not, approach the stretching exercises slowly and carefully. If you'll exercise your patience and your sense of humor when you do the stretches, you shouldn't have any problems.

Q. Should pregnant women stretch?

A. Generally, regular exercise during pregnancy is essential for the health of the mother and her baby. Stretching exercises, particularly those that emphasize conditioning the pelvic region, are especially advantageous for the pregnant woman. Positions that elevate the legs are also helpful. It is usually considered unwise to begin a challenging exercise program after you are already pregnant. So, if you are pregnant and regular exercise is something new for you, use your common sense in the stretches, and save the more difficult exercises until after your baby is born. However, if you were already exercising regularly before your pregnancy, you will probably benefit from most of the stretching exercises in this book. Adjust them to fit your capabilities as your pregnancy progresses. During the last trimester, you will probably find some positions especially soothing, while others may become impossible. No matter what your level of fitness was prior to your pregnancy, consult your physician about stretching and, with his approval, exercise slowly and carefully. Let your body be your guide.

Q. Should children do the stretching exercises?

A. Children are constantly stretching during play. Their muscles and joints are usually supple and flexible. From time to time, you'll probably find your children wanting to join you as you stretch. Even if they do express interest, treat their participation casually and keep it on a "play" level. Resist the urge to compete with your child: stretching should be fun for adults as well as for children.

* * *

Perhaps best of all, stretching feels good. Its everyday rewards are noticeable, and if you're on a sports training schedule, it's an ingredient that shouldn't be left out in your pursuit of the winning advantage.

4

Warmups

"I used to just jump out of my car and start running, and I used to have a lot more running injuries then, too. Now I warm up with stretching exercises before each run," says James McNair, M.D., a veteran of thirteen years of running. The doctor takes his running seriously, too, having competed in over twenty marathons, and posting a personal-best under three hours. Dr. McNair is the director of the Little Rock Human Performance Center, a holistic health clinic that through individual evaluation and education hopes to improve a client's overall health. Warm-up exercises play an important role in any exercise prescription administered by Dr. McNair, who believes that "consistency is an important part of a stretching exercise program, and stretching is a regular part of my own training."

Taking ten minutes to prepare your body for a run can be considered good preventive therapy. Weak or inflexible muscles tear relatively easily. This tearing may occur in the main body of the muscle when a sudden stretch follows a maximum contraction. The tear may also occur at the muscle's tendon connection, or at the tendon-bone attachment. When short, inflexible muscles surround a joint, they set the stage for a torn ligament, tendon, muscle or dislocation.

Fortunately, being a runner doesn't mean you have to play a game of muscle-tear roulette. You can greatly enhance your chances of enjoying injury-free running by incorporating a warm-up into your training. Warm-up exercises prepare you physically for a training run. Later, if you compete, the warmup can keep you relaxed and your thoughts focused on the event in the tense pre-race minutes.

1. Growing Taller

1. Stand with your feet slightly apart, arms to the sides. Lift the chest, contract the buttocks, tuck the tail under. Lift the kneecaps.
2. Balance equally on both feet. Keep the face and abdomen relaxed and imagine the entire body growing up from the feet, then feel the waist thinning as the stretch continues up from the hips. The extension grows from the ground up, so don't pull or lift the head. This exercise is good preparation for the standing stretches that follow.
Benefits: Firms buttocks and thighs, expands chest. Increases awareness of body's alignment or lack of alignment.

2. Side Stretch

1. Stand with the feet slightly apart. Grasp a towel or a stick between your hands and continue to "grow tall" as you extend your arms up and stretch.
2. Exhale, bend at the hips to the right. Keep arms and legs straight. Hold for five to ten seconds. Don't allow the upper body to twist, so keep the buttock muscles contracted to stabilize the exercise. Reverse.
Benefits: Good for waist, legs, arms and shoulders.

3. Back Extender

1. Face a table, ledge or sink. Holding the ledge, walk back until the legs are perpendicular to the floor. Form a right angle with hips; keep back and arms straight. Lift the kneecaps, and keep the face and neck loose.
2. Exhale, lift the tail slightly, extending the back more. Hold for fifteen to twenty seconds and release the pose by walking in. Build up to one to two minutes.
Benefits: Great stretch for legs, back and shoulders.

4. Kneeling Back Extender

1. If your legs are stiff, try this variation of the Back Extender. Kneel in front of a sturdy chair, hold your wrists or elbows, place elbows on chair.
2. Exhale, extend the back to a maximum stretch, with knees slightly apart. Hold for fifteen to twenty seconds.
Benefits: Loosens shoulders and back.

1. Growing Taller

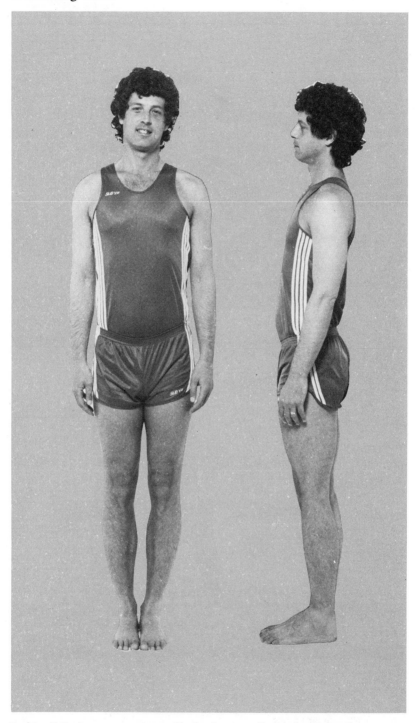

Growing Taller increases awareness of body alignment. Do it in front of a mirror.

2. Side Stretch

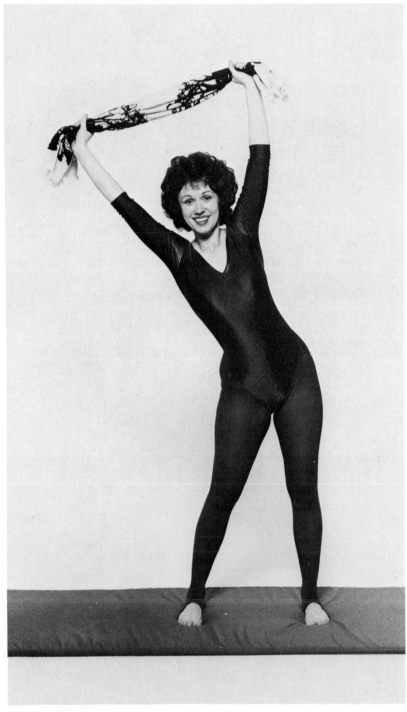

Use a towel to do Side Stretch.

3. Back Extender

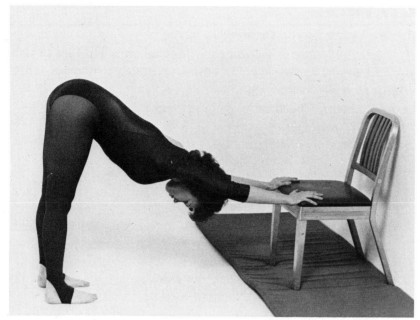

To do Back Extender, use a table, ledge, sink, or chair; keep your back straight.

4. Kneeling Back Extender

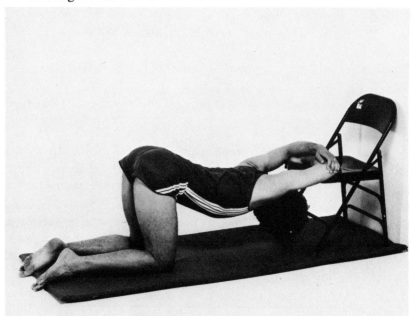

The Kneeling Back Extender is good for a stiff back.

5. Leg Stretch

1. Face a chair and do Growing Taller.

2. Exhale, place right heel on chair, extend arms and toes straight up. Lift the kneecaps, keeping both legs straight. Hold for ten to fifteen seconds. Switch legs.

3. As an exercise becomes easier, use a higher ledge and hold longer, building to one minute.
Benefits: Stretches hamstrings.

6. Twisting Leg Stretch

1. Assume Leg Stretch position with arms extended horizontally.

2. Exhale, keep legs straight as you turn trunk to right, hold for a few breaths, then turn left. Change legs and repeat.
Benefits: Good warmup for back and legs.

7. Bent Knee Leg Stretch

1. Stand with right side to chair. Turn out both legs from hips, place right heel on chair.

2. Exhale, bend left knee, right leg stays straight. Straighten your back and place hands at waist. Hold for fifteen to twenty seconds; change legs.
Benefits: Good hamstring stretch variation if legs are stiff.

8. Triangle

1. Stand with feet 3 - 3½ feet apart. Turn left foot in thirty degrees, right leg out ninety degrees. Stretch arms out to side. Align the feet with the right foot on an imaginary line that bisects the left foot.

2. Exhale, bend from the hips to the right. Keep the legs straight, push right hip forward, bring left hip and shoulder slightly back. Extend trunk straight out to the right so that the right side of waist stretches in line with right leg.

3. Turn chest toward the ceiling, not to the floor. In the beginning, rest the right hand on the leg. Hold for fifteen to twenty seconds. Exhale, come up from the hips. Change sides.
Benefits: Excellent stretch for feet, legs, hips and back.

5. Leg Stretch

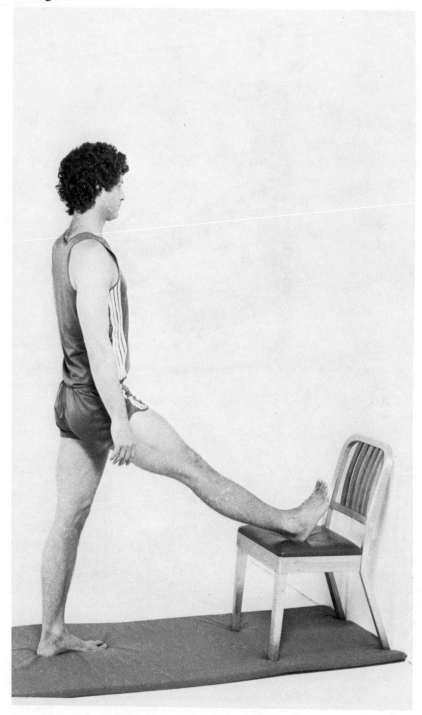

Leg Stretch works the hamstrings.

6. Twisting Leg Stretch

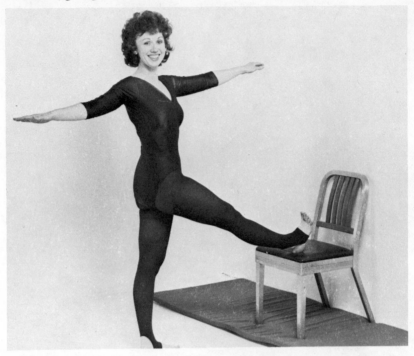

In Twisting Leg Stretch you turn at the trunk. It's a good warmup for the legs and back.

7. Bent Knee Leg Stretch

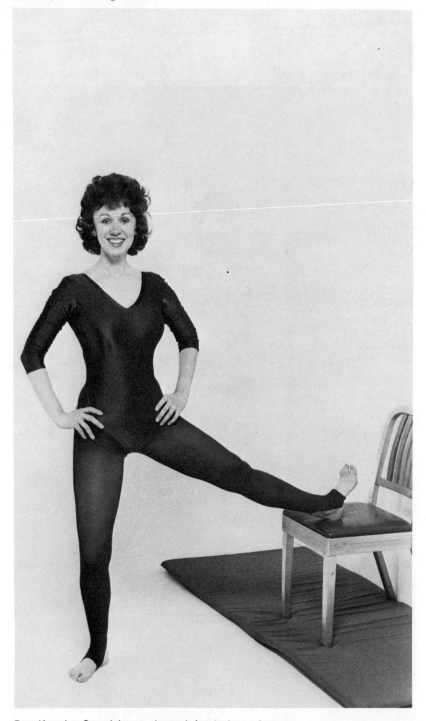

Bent Knee Leg Stretch is a good stretch for the hamstrings.

8. Triangle

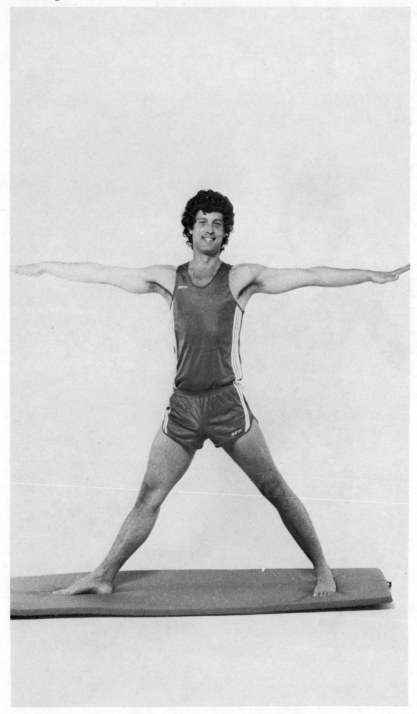

Note symmetry of body to start Triangle.

8. Triangle (CONT'D.)

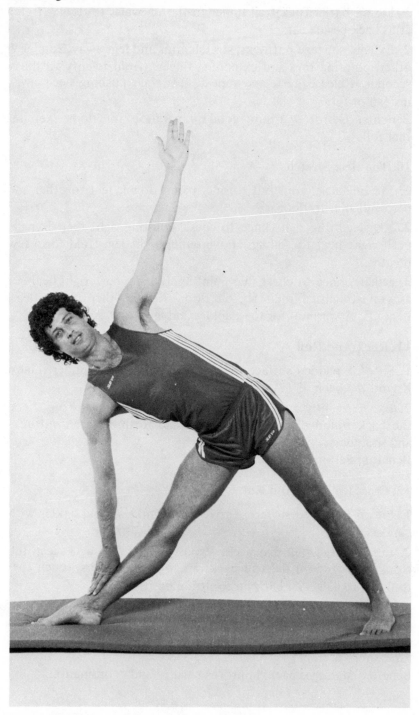

Keep legs straight when bringing right arm to right foot.

9. Growing Longer

1. Lie on back. Tuck trail under to flatten waist to floor. Stretch arms back beside ears.

2. Exhale, squeeze buttocks, stretch arms and legs away from each other, pointing toes and extending fingers. Hold twenty to thirty seconds. Release, rest, and repeat, this time pushing heels away instead of toes.

Benefits: Gentle warmup; good preparation for floor exercises that follow.

10. Toe-Heel Stretch

1. Lie on back, arms out to side, palms down, feet together and perpendicular to floor.

2. Exhale, bring right knee to chest, pointing right toes. Exhale, push right heel to ceiling, straightening right leg. Hold for a few breaths.

3. Exhale, knee to chest, toe pointing. Exhale, push right heel out as you straighten right leg on floor. Repeat, then change legs.

Benefits: A warmup for toes, ankles and legs.

11. Rock And Roll

1. Sit on a padded surface. Bend knees, hold wrists under thighs. Round the back.

2. Exhale, gently roll back on spine. Inhale, rock back up. Keep the back rounded as you rock back and forth between buttocks and shoulders.

Benefits: Self-massage for the back.

12. Cross-leg Rock And Roll

1. Sit on a padded surface. Cross legs at ankles, hold ankles with hands.

2. Inhale, straighten the back. Exhale, round the back, lean the trunk forward. Inhale, roll backward onto shoulders, touch toes to floor. Exhale, roll back up to sitting position.

3. Cycle is repeated as follows: Inhale, sit up straight. Exhale, bend forward. Inhale, roll back. Exhale, roll up. Pause at any stage during the cycle for a deeper stretch or simply keep the momentum going.

Benefits: Massages back, improves balance and coordination.

9. Growing Longer

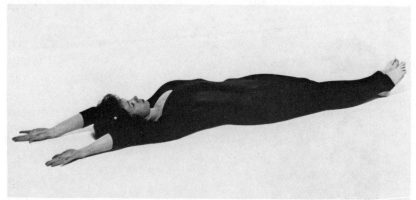

Lying on your back, extend your arms and s-t-r-e-t-c-h. That's Growing Longer.

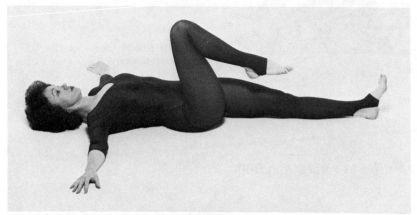

Bring right knee to chest to start Toe-Heel Stretch.

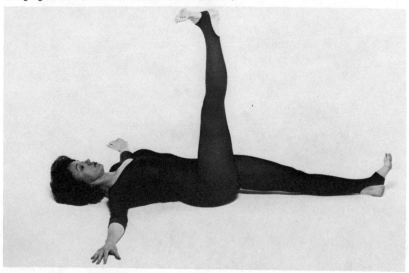

Then extend the right leg up.

11. Rock And Roll

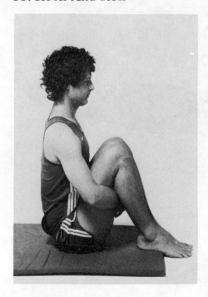

Rock And Roll requires a padded surface, but not Buddy Holly.

12. Cross Leg Rock And Roll

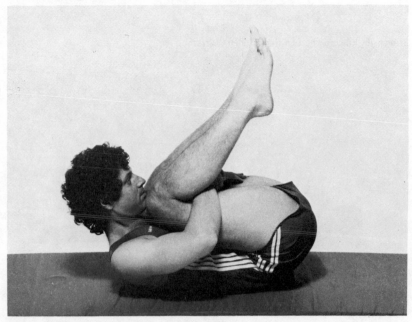

Roll back onto your spine and then rock back up.

12. Cross Leg Rock And Roll (CONT'D.)

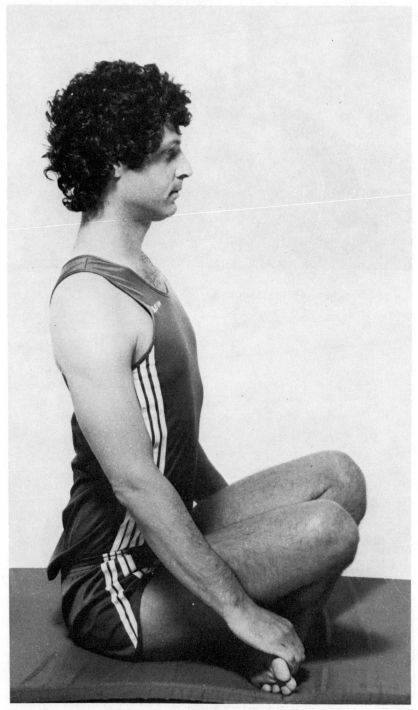

Cross-Leg Rock And Roll calls for some fancy footwork.

(CONT'D NEXT PAGE)

12. Cross Leg Rock And Roll (CONT'D.)

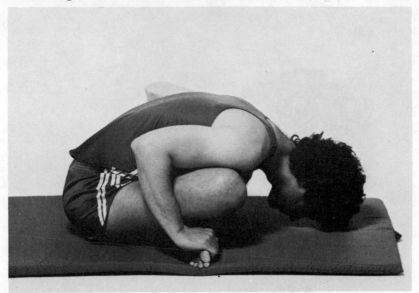

Lean your trunk forward before rolling back.

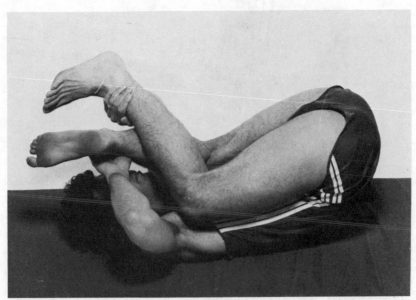

Now roll onto your back as far as you can, and return.

13. Chorus Line

1. Lie on back, arms out to side forming a "T," palms down. Put feet perpendicular and together. Flatten waist to floor. Bend right knee, place right foot on left knee.

2. Exhale, roll right knee over to left. Keep back relaxed, right shoulder and both palms on floor. Gently turn head to right. Hold ten to fifteen seconds. Reverse.
Benefits: Loosens spine and shoulders.

14. Heel in Toe Twist

1. Lie on back as in Chorus Line. Wedge right heel between left big toe and next toe.

2. Exhale, roll right leg and hip over to left, without moving right heel position. Right shoulder and both palms flat. Gently turn head to right. Hold ten to fifteen seconds. Change legs.
Benefits: Gentle warmup for spine, shoulders.

15. Puppy Stretch

1. Kneel on pad with knees apart, lean forward and walk hands out as far as possible. Hands, shoulders, hips and knees should be aligned.

2. Exhale, draw hips back toward heels, keeping hands on floor. Arms straight, with head resting on floor.
Benefits: Elongates back; good preparation for Downward Dog.

16. Downward Dog

1. Kneel on all fours, form a table with your back by placing arms and thighs perpendicular to floor. Keep hands as wide apart as shoulders, toes turned under.

2. Exhale, straighten legs. Lift heels and buttocks high toward ceiling. Press down on the hands; stretch the shoulders and hips away from the hands in a straight line that points to the ceiling. Keep this stretch as you press heels down. Lift kneecaps, straighten legs. Hold twenty to thirty seconds, build to one to three minutes.
Benefits: Excellent overall warmup; stretches entire backside of body.

17. Groin Stretch

1. Squat, extend left knee back, balancing on knee, lower leg and foot.

2. Exhale, release tension in groin, push both hips forward. Rest hands on right knee, lift chest, drop shoulders. Extend arms out for balance. Hold fifteen to twenty seconds. Change legs.
Benefits: Loosens hips, groin.

18. Chair Groin Stretch

1. Face chair. Place right foot on chair with knee bent, hands on right knee.

2. Exhale, sink both hips down toward the chair. Push left heel down to keep left leg straight. Keep the back as straight as possible with shoulders back. Hold ten to fifteen seconds. Change legs.
Benefits: Loosens groin and hamstrings.

19. Beginning Lateral Stretch

1. Place feet 4 - 4½ feet apart. Turn left foot in thirty degrees, right leg out ninety degrees. Align feet as in Triangle. Stretch arms out, palms down.

2. Exhale, bend right knee in line with right foot. Don't allow the knee to lean in: keep outer edge of knee pointing to little toe. Lower right leg is perpendicular to floor. Left leg is straight with knee locked.

3. Exhale, stretch from hip to the right. Right hand holds inside right lower leg. Stretch left arm straight up. Chest and abdomen face opposite wall, not floor. Hold twenty to thirty seconds. Change sides.
Benefits: Improves stretch in legs, groin and hips. Good preparation for Extended Lateral.

20. Extended Lateral Stretch

1. Place feet 4 - 4½ feet apart. Turn left foot in thirty degrees, right leg out ninety degrees. Align feet as in Triangle. Stretch arms out, palms down.

2. Exhale, bend right knee to a right angle. Place right thigh parallel to floor, lower leg perpendicular to floor. Bent knee stays in line with foot: don't let the knee lean in; see Beginning Lateral Stretch.

3. Exhale, stretch right side of body from right hip, extending waist along right thigh. Right palm or fingertips on floor beside foot, left arm straight and stretching over left ear. Push right hip through, turn chest and abdomen from hips to face ceiling. Hold fifteen to twenty seconds. Reverse.
Benefits: Intense stretch for legs, groin, hips and waist.

21. Wall Hang

1. Stand with back about a foot away from wall, feet ten to twelve inches apart, toes turned in. Place back on wall, fingers in hip joint.

2. Exhale, treat the back as a single unit and bend from the hips.

Tip the pelvis to lift the sitting bones higher up the wall. Extend the spine horizontally until it feels parallel with the floor.

3. Use your hands at the waist to check for an indention. If the bony parts of the spine are protruding, lift the torso higher until you do create the "flat back." (As you become more flexible, you'll feel the concave spine, or "flat back," at a different angle.)

4. When you've reached your maximum bend from the hips with a "flat back," round the back to complete the exercise. Keep the kneecaps raised, the abdomen relaxed. Hold ten to fifteen seconds. Tuck the tail under and roll up wall to release.
Benefits: Stretches the legs and the back.

22. Roll Down Hang

1. Stand with feet about one foot apart and parallel.

2. Exhale, tuck the chin under, round the shoulders and bend forward, hanging from the hips. Raise kneecaps, straighten legs. Hang arms loosely. Hold ten to twenty seconds. Release by coming up with a round back.
Benefits: Stretches hamstrings, back.

23. Intense Hanging Stretch

1. Stand with feet about one foot apart and parallel. Squeeze the buttocks, tuck the tail under. Stretch the arms up, bend the elbows, hold elbows or wrists.

2. Exhale, with a flat back; bend at hips as in Wall Hang. Lift sitting bones toward ceiling. Stretch elbows out to form a parallel line with the floor. Continue to bend and hang from the hips.

3. Keep abdomen and face relaxed. Lift and widen the hips. Raise kneecaps, straighten legs. Hold twenty to thirty seconds. Release arms, round the back and roll up. (As the back muscles strengthen, you will be able to come up with a "flat back.")
Benefits: Stretches hamstrings, loosens back.

24. Runner's Stretch

1. Squat with right foot about one foot in front of left, hands beside right foot. Point both feet straight ahead.

2. Exhale, straighten legs and arms. Lift kneecaps and tail toward ceiling. (If you can't keep fingertips on floor, use books or a ledge under hands.) Hold fifteen to twenty seconds. Change legs.
Benefits: Loosens hips and legs.

25. Prone Back Leg Lift

1. Lie face down, your chin on the floor with arms along body, palms down. Point toes with legs and feet together.

2. Exhale, squeeze buttocks, lift right leg, keeping both pelvic bones against the floor. Hold five to ten seconds. Change legs.

3. As your back strengthens, try both legs. First turn hands up and slip them under groin. Exhale, lift both legs, keeping feet together, buttocks firm. Hold five to ten seconds.
Benefits: Strengthens lower back.

26. Prone Body Lift

1. Lie face down, legs and feet together, toes pointed. Stretch arms forward along ears, palms down.

2. Exhale, contract buttocks and lift arms, head, chest and legs. Hold for ten to fifteen seconds. Vary this exercise by stretching arms to the side.
Benefits: Strengthens lower back.

27. The Bow

1. Lie face down, bend knees, hold ankles behind your back with corresponding hands. Knees may separate but keep lower legs parallel.

2. Exhale, simultaneously lift feet, knees and chest. Squeeze buttocks. Hold for ten to fifteen seconds. (As you improve the exercise, the knees can be brought closer together.)
Benefits: Brings elasticity to spine, strengthens lower back and stretches quadriceps.

28. Yoga Warmup — Sun Salute

1. Stand in Growing Taller. Turn palms out.

2. Inhale, stretch arms overhead. Keep buttocks contracted, tail tucked under.

3. Exhale, bend from hips with a flat back, do Intense Hanging Stretch. If you have a weak back, do Roll Down Hang.

4. Hands are beside feet now, fingers pointing forward. Bend knees if necessary.

5. Inhale, Groin Stretch with left foot back, toes turned under.

6. Hold breath, take right foot back for Push-Up position. Firm buttocks, flatten shoulder blades.

7. Exhale, (spine recoils as you bend elbows and knees), lift buttocks. Touch knees, chest, and chin simultaneously to floor.

8. Inhale, Upward Dog.

9. Exhale, Downward Dog.

10. Inhale, Groin Stretch, left leg forward.

11. Exhale, Intense Hanging Stretch.

12. Inhale, Growing Taller. Come up with a flat back or by tucking tail under and rolling up. Repeat with right leg back in step 5, right leg forward in step 11.

Benefits: Brings flexibility to spine and legs, stretches and strengthens arms and shoulders. Develops coordination and breath control.

13. Chorus Line

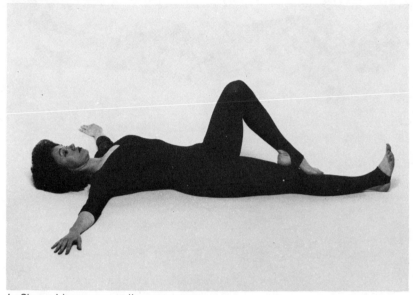

In Chorus Line you get to lie on your back.

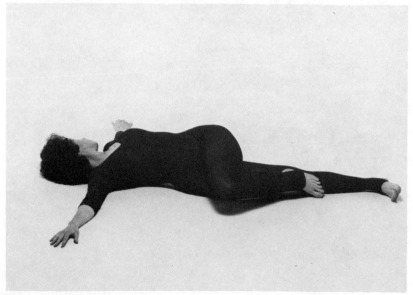

This exercise loosens the spine and shoulders.

14. Heel In Toe Twist

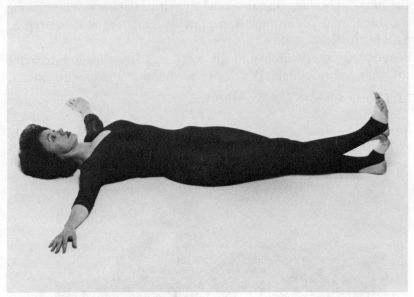

You roll your hips in the Heel-in-toe Twist.

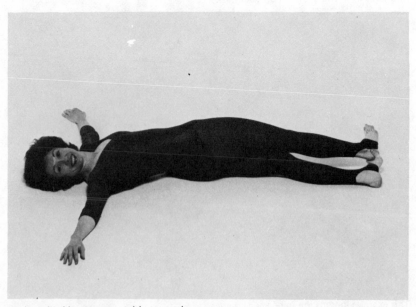

Wedge a heel between your big toe and next toe.

15. Puppy Stretch

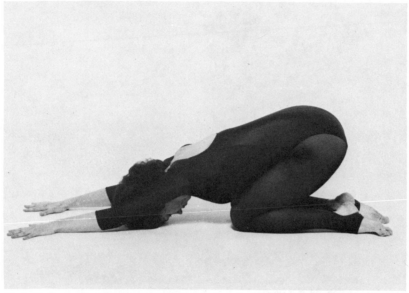

By doing Puppy Stretch, your prayers for an elongated back will be answered.

16. Downward Dog

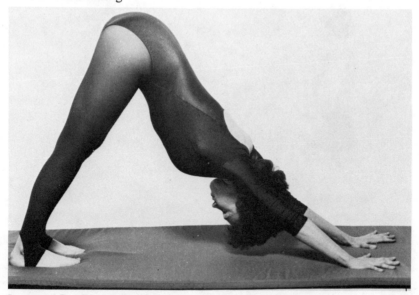

Downward Dog forms an inverted V. It stretches the entire backside of body.

17. Groin Stretch

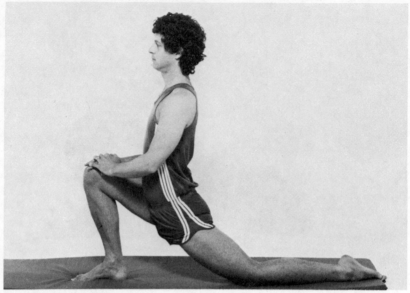

Groin Stretch does what it says.

18. Chair Groin Stretch

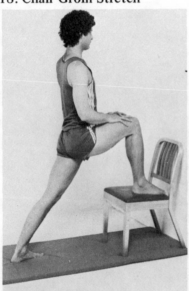

With hands on a knee, in Chair Groin Stretch, sink hips to chair.

19. Beginning Lateral Stretch

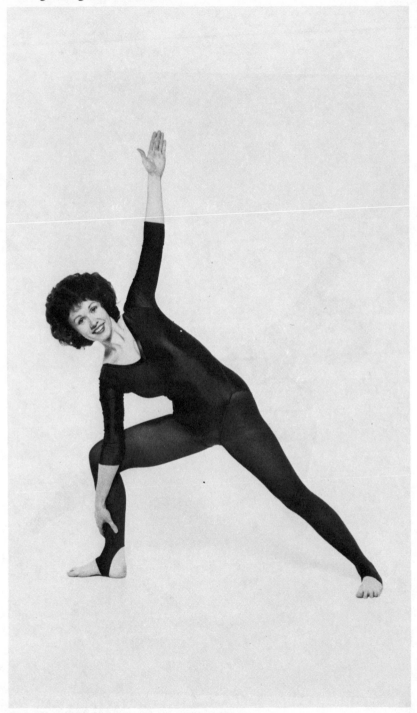

Beginning Lateral Stretch works legs, groin and hips.

20. Extended Lateral Stretch

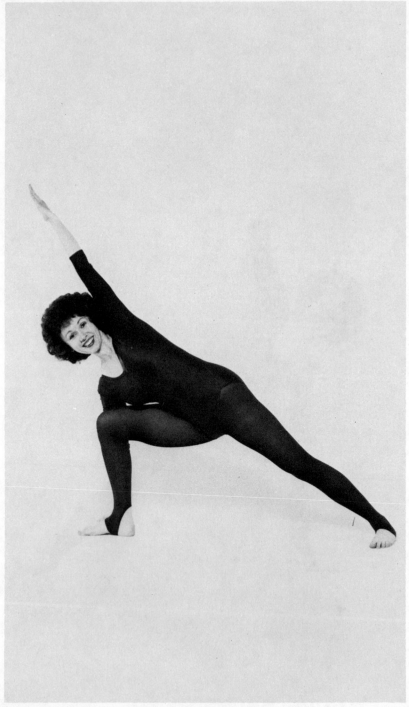

Note how the arm and leg in Extended Lateral Stretch are in line.

21. Wall Hang

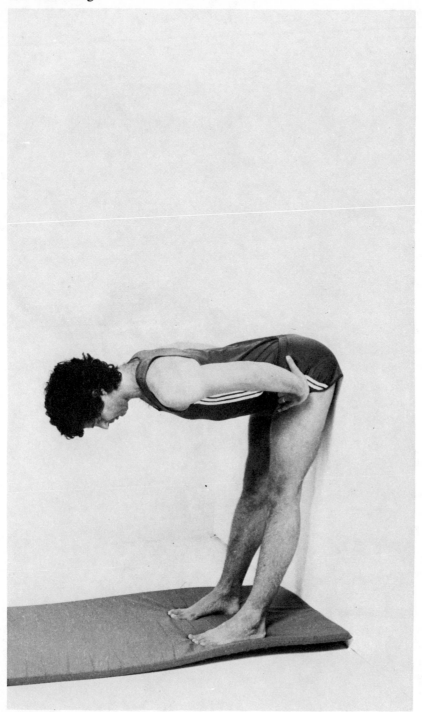

Stand with your back about a foot away from the wall for Wall Hang.

(CONT'D NEXT PAGE)

21. Wall Hang (CONT'D.)

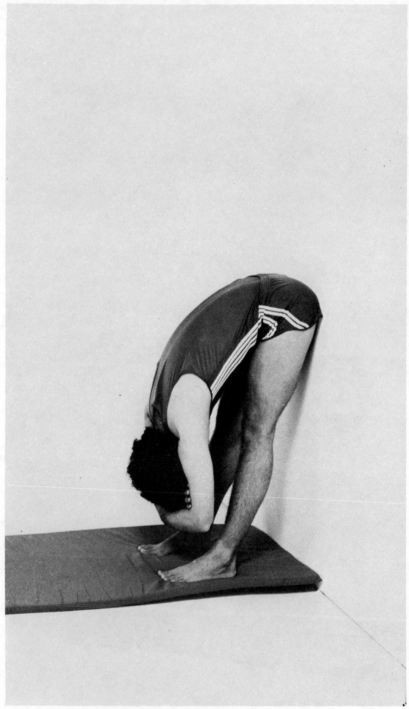

Keep your back flat when you bend at the waist.

22. Roll Down Hang

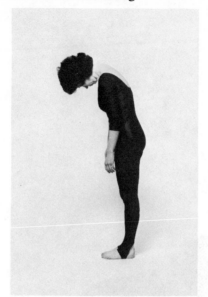

Tuck chin and let arms hang in Roll Down Hang.

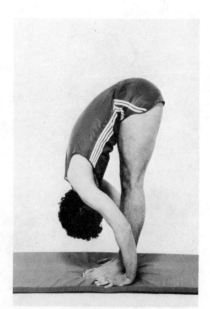

Roll Down stretches the hamstrings and back.

23. Intense Hanging Stretch

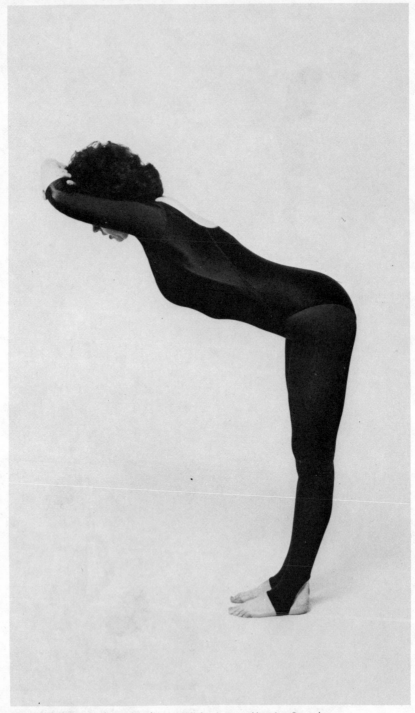

Squeeze your buttocks and tuck your tail for Intense Hanging Stretch.

23. Intense Hanging Stretch (CONT'D.)

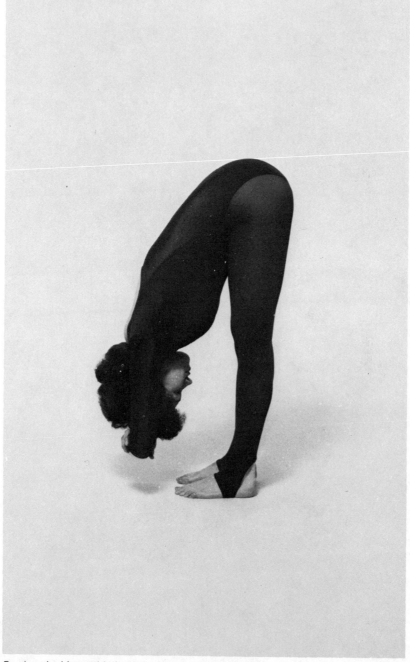

Bend at the hips and hold for twenty to thirty seconds.

24. Runner's Stretch

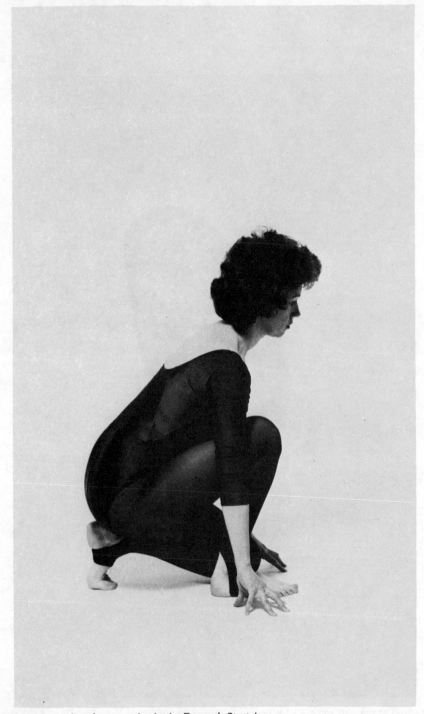

Assume a sprinter's pose to begin the Runner's Stretch.

24. Runner's Stretch (CONT'D.)

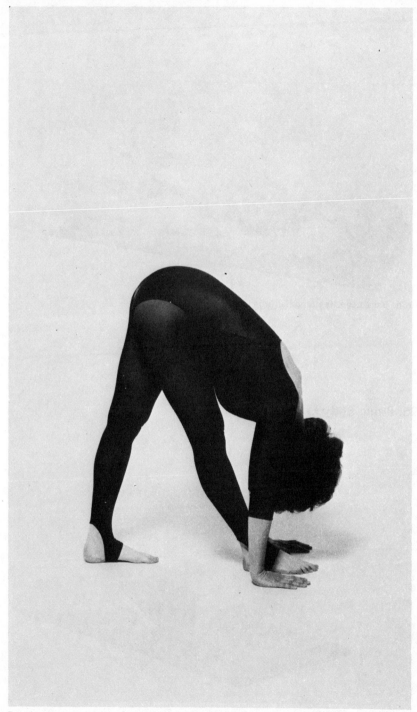

Exhale, then straighten legs and arms. Use a book if you can't keep fingers on floor.

25. Prone Back Leg Lift

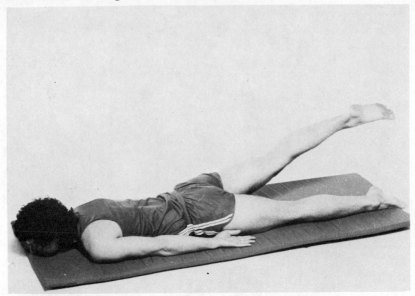

Prone Back Leg Lift strengthens the lower back.

26. Prone Body Lift

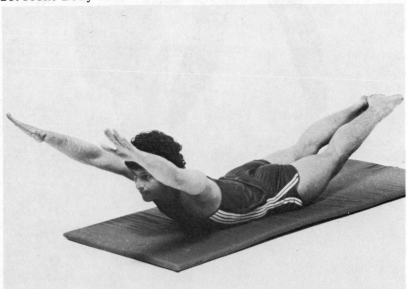

With your body straight in Prone Body Lift, lift your arms, chest and legs.

27. The Bow

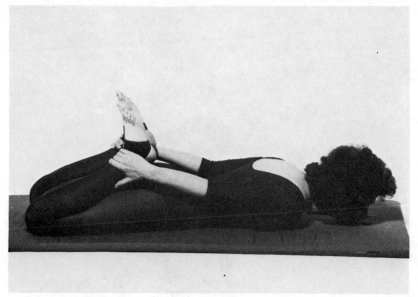

Grasp your ankles with your hands in The Bow.

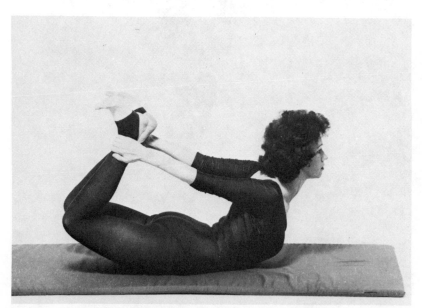

Now lift your chest off the floor and tighten buttocks.

28. Yoga Warmup - Sun Salute

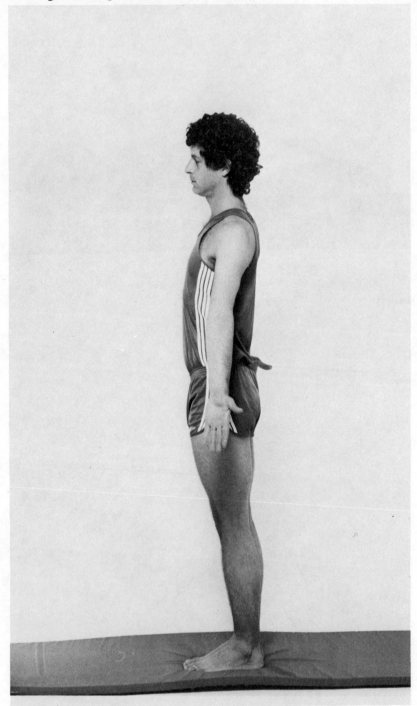

This yoga warmup is called Sun Salute. It develops coordination and breath control.

28. Yoga Warmup - Sun Salute (CONT'D.)

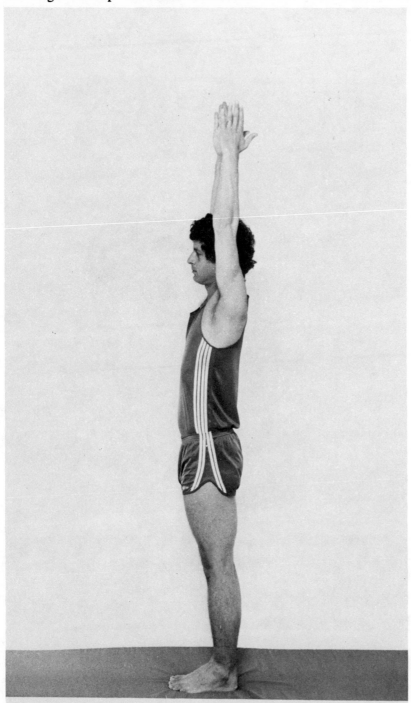

Stand straight and raise your arms over your head.

(CONT'D NEXT PAGE)

28. Yoga Warmup - Sun Salute (CONT'D.)

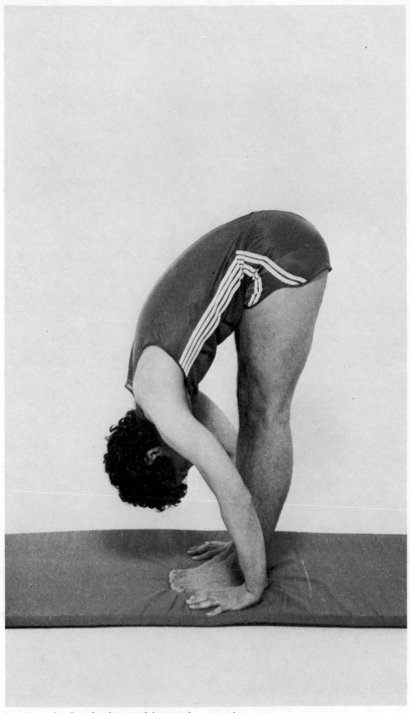

Bend at waist, keeping legs straight; touch nose to knees.

28. Yoga Warmup - Sun Salute (CONT'D.)

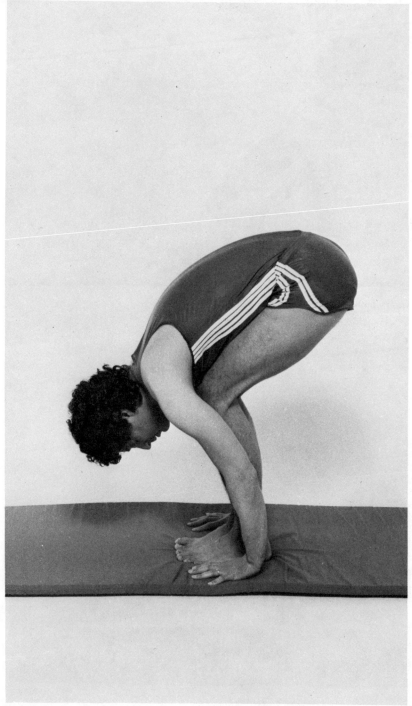

Bend knees if need be to touch hands to floor next to feet.

(CONT'D NEXT PAGE)

28. Yoga Warmup - Sun Salute (CONT'D.)

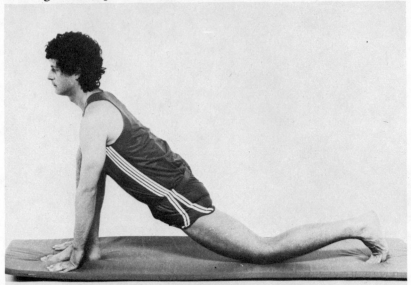

Assume push-up position, legs bent at knee.

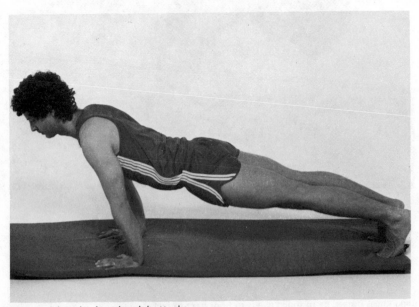

Now straighten back and tuck buttocks.

28. Yoga Warmup - Sun Salute (CONT'D.)

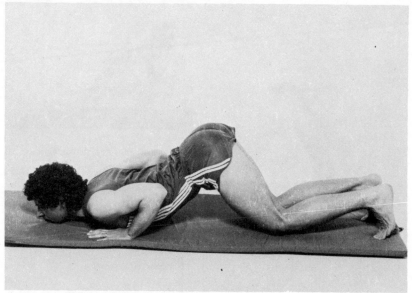

Exhale and touch chin, chest and knees to floor simultaneously.

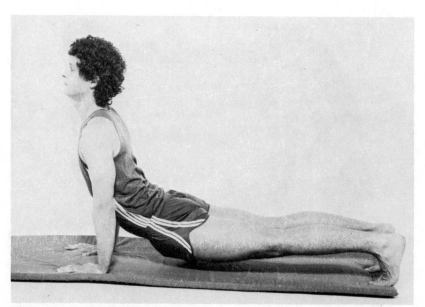

Inhale and go to Upward Dog.

(CONT'D NEXT PAGE)

28. Yoga Warmup - Sun Salute (CONT'D.)

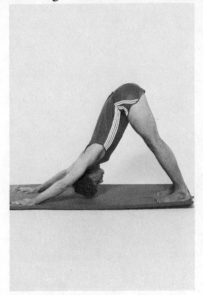

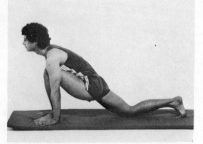

Then extend a leg and stretch a groin.

Exhale and go to Downward Dog.

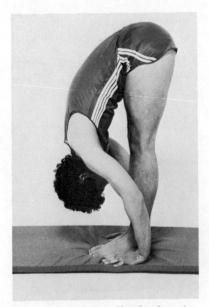

Exhale and do Intense Hanging Stretch.

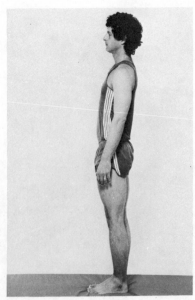

Finish with Growing Taller.

5

Feet and Legs

The maintenance of feet and legs is essential to good running. The weight of your entire upper body is transferred from the hips through your thighs to the knees and on to the ankles and feet via the shins. Your weight is then distributed to the twenty-six bones in each foot.

The muscles of your legs and buttocks are the largest and strongest muscles in your body. Those who run on a regular basis firm and strengthen their leg muscles. During the early stages of a running program, this improvement in muscle tone can be an encouraging stimulus to your running commitment. The thighs change from flab to muscle, the calf muscles appear stronger and the legs look longer and leaner. But as the months and miles go by, the legs, while still strong, get tight and inflexible. Running overdevelops the muscles along the back of your legs, while relatively weakening the muscles in the front of your legs.

This muscle stiffening is usually felt in the knees, lower legs or lower back. The hamstring muscles extend from the buttocks to below the back of the knees, so inflexibility in these muscles can inhibit mobility in the hips and/or knee joints. The gastrocnemius muscle of the calf also affects body alignment and knee joint fluidity. Lower back pain can result when movement usually done by the legs is by necessity absorbed by the back. An immobile, stiff knee can be uncomfortable and set the stage for injuries. The strongest tendon in the body—the Achilles—controls the plantar and dorsi-flexion of the foot. If this tendon is stiff and inflexible, painful irritation and inflammation may result.

Several factors can contribute to maximum muscle and joint efficiency in the legs and feet of runners: good shoes, the correction of any structural imbalance, and a regular stretching program.

The exercises in this chapter will cover stretching. By stretching regularly, you'll strengthen the shins and the front thighs, while stretching the feet and the backs of the legs.

To a great extent, your feet and legs control your running. They get you on the road, and then carry you over it. When they operate at a maximum level of efficiency, you travel in style, and pain-free.

1. Ledge Stretch

1. Face a ledge that's about chest-high. Stand an arm's length away and hold the ledge with both hands. Tuck the tail under.

2. Exhale, bend the elbows, keep the body straight, heels on floor. Hold for a few breaths.

3. Now exhale, straighten arms and rock back on heels, allowing buttocks to fall back. Hold for a few breaths; repeat.
Benefits: Stretches Achilles tendon and calves.

2. Straight Leg Calf Stretch

1. Face a wall. Right toes on wall, right heel on floor. Position left foot three feet back of and facing wall. Place hands on wall, which is opposite shoulders. Lift left heel.

2. Exhale, press left heel down, press hands against wall, straightening arms and moving chest and shoulders slightly back. Tuck tail under. Hold ten to fifteen seconds. Change legs.
Benefits: Good stretch for calves and ankles.

3. Bent Knee Calf Stretch

1. Face wall as in Straight Leg Calf Stretch. Back heel up.

2. Exhale, bend front knee forward toward wall, simultaneously pressing back heel down. Expand chest, keep tail tucked under. Hold five to ten seconds. Reverse leg positions.
Benefits: Stretches calves.

4. The Wall Chair

1. Stand with back to wall, about a foot away. Lean back on wall. Feet are eight to twelve inches apart and parallel.

2. Exhale, bend the knees and slide the back down the wall. Tuck the tail under, press the waist to wall. Keep knees in line with feet, hands on knees or extend arms up alongside ears. Hold ten to fifteen seconds, building to one minute. Release by straightening

legs, sliding back up wall.
Benefits: Strengthens quadriceps.

5. Invisible Chair

1. Stand with feet slightly apart and parallel. Lift the arms beside ears. Tuck the tail under.
2. Exhale, bend knees, keeping knees in line with feet. Try not to lean forward. Sit in the chair for a few breaths.
Benefits: Strengthens quadriceps, improves balance and sense of humor.

6. The Dancer

1. Stand inside a doorway. Hold the doorjamb an arm's length away. Place the feet about three to four feet apart, toes turning out. Tuck tail under.
2. Exhale, bend knees until thighs are parallel to floor. Knees stop directly over heels, lower legs are perpendicular to floor. Keep trunk erect, knees moving back. Hold ten to fifteen seconds; repeat.
Benefits: Tones calves and thighs.

7. Proud Warrior

1. Place feet 4 - 4½ feet apart, arms stretched horizontally. Turn left foot in thirty degrees, right leg out ninety degrees. Tuck tail under. Align feet as in Triangle.
2. Exhale, bend right knee until lower leg forms a perpendicular line with floor. Right thigh is parallel to floor. Outer edge of right knee points to right little toe. (Right knee should never fall in.) Keep torso erect, left leg straight. Hold twenty to thirty seconds. Reverse.
Benefits: Stretches and shapes the calves, thighs and hamstrings.

8. Squat Challenge I

1. Kneel on all fours, toes turned under.
2. Exhale, sit back on heels. Keep back erect, tail tucked under. Hold for a few seconds, then do Squat Challenge II.

9. Squat Challenge II

1. Exhale, lift knees, keep thighs parallel to floor, and buttocks still on heels. Stretch arms out in front for balance. Back stays erect. Continue to Squat Challenge III.

10. Squat Challenge III

1. Exhale, press heels to floor, keep knees together. Hold ten seconds; reverse cycle. (Place a book under the heels if they don't touch the floor.)
Benefits: Squat cycle stretches Achilles tendon, strengthens feet and legs.

11. Sitting Challenge I

1. Kneel on all fours on a padded surface. Place knees and feet together.
2.Exhale, slowly walk hands back as you sit on your heels. Tuck the tail under, rest the hands on thighs, keep the back erect. The feet can be slightly separated, but they should point straight back. (If this is difficult, try sitting with a pillow between feet and buttocks.) Be very careful in any sitting exercise that involves bending the knees.
Benefits: Stretches feet, ankles and legs.

12. Sitting Challenge II

1. Sit in position of Sitting Challenge I. Lift buttocks, bring the feet wider apart.
2. Exhale, tuck tail under as you gently lower buttocks to floor. (Sometimes, using your hands to separate thigh and calf muscles will facilitate this sitting position.) In the beginning, sit on a pillow. The knees may separate, but work toward keeping them together. Hold for a few seconds; build up to thirty seconds and then one minute.
Benefits: Loosens calf and thigh muscles, increases flexibility in feet.

13. Sitting Challenge III (Proceed to III only if II is easy.)

1. Sit in position of Sitting Challenge II. Place several pillows behind you.
2. Exhale, gently lower yourself back on your elbows. Lift buttocks slightly and tuck tail under. Slowly lower back to pillows. Flatten waist. For the novice, knees usually separate, but eventually you should learn to keep them together. Hold for a few breaths; come up by using elbows.
Benefits: Stretches feet, legs and back.

14. Sitting Challenge IV (When III becomes easy, continue to IV.)

1. Sit in position of Sitting Challenge II.

2. Exhale, using elbows for support as in III, gradually lower back to floor. Lift buttocks slightly and tuck tail under. Bring knees together. Stretch arms back along ears, palms up. Keep stretching arms as you flatten waist to floor. Hold for a few breaths, come up by using elbows.
Benefits: Intense stretch for feet, ankles, legs and back.

15. Sitting Challenge V

1. Sit in position of Sitting Challenge II. Straighten the right leg then bring right knee to chest, supporting back of thigh with hands. Sit erect.

2. Exhale, straighten right leg toward ceiling, pushing heel away. Hold for a few breaths, change sides. (If the back rounds, try using a towel or belt around the foot. Hold the ends of the towel with your hands, pull gently on the towel while lifting the chest to straighten the back.) Work toward holding the ankle or the foot.
Benefits: Intense leg stretch.

16. Resting Leg Stretch

1. Lie on left side, rest on left elbow, support the head with the hand. Elbow, shoulders, hips and feet form a straight line. Turn right leg toward ceiling, bend the right knee, hold right big toe with right hand. Left leg is straight, foot flat.

2. Exhale, straighten leg toward ceiling. Do not allow right hip to roll back. (If the leg will not straighten with the toe hold, try this same exercise with right hand on floor.) Hold ten to fifteen seconds. Change sides.
Benefits: Stretches hamstrings, loosens hips.

17. Resting Leg Lift I

1. Lie in Resting Leg Stretch position.

2. Exhale, push balls of feet away and lift straight legs, keeping feet together. Don't roll back on buttocks. Hold ten to fifteen seconds, repeat. Reverse.
Benefits: Stretches and strengthens hips and thighs.

18. Resting Leg Lift II

1. Lie on left side in Resting Leg Lift I. Bend right knee, place right foot on floor beside left knee. Roll right hip slightly forward.
2. Exhale, press ball of left foot away and lift straight leg. Hold ten to fifteen seconds; repeat. Change sides.
Benefits: Tones and strengthens inner thigh.

19. Archer

1. Sit in the Right Angle (p.87). Lean forward and hold big toes.
2. Exhale, bend the right leg, draw right knee back toward body. Left leg is straight.
3. Exhale, straighten right leg out to side.
4. Exhale, swing straight leg up, lifting it close to right ear. Release to floor. Repeat this cycle five to ten times on both sides. (Hold ankle if necessary.)
Benefits: Loosens legs and hips, strengthens arms.

20. Thigh Stretch

1. Get on all fours, place knees and feet as wide apart as hips, keeping lower legs parallel. Balance on knees with arms stretched out in front. Squeeze buttocks, tuck tail under.
2. Exhale, lean entire body slightly back, keeping tail tucked. Hold five to ten seconds, repeat.
Benefits: Excellent thigh strengthener.

21. Supported Runner's Balance

1. Face a chair or ledge. Do the Back Extender.
2. Exhale, lift right leg, keeping it straight and pointing ball of foot. Keep buttocks level, stretch leg up from hip without allowing right hip to lift up or left hip to drop. Both legs are straight, knee-caps lifted. Hold ten to fifteen seconds. Change sides.
Benefits: Strengthens and stretches legs. Good preparation for Runner's Balance.

22. Runner's Balance

1. Stand with feet parallel and 4 - 4½ feet apart. Inhale, stretch arms up along ears, keep shoulders down. Turn left foot in thirty degrees, right leg out ninety degrees. Align feet as in Triangle. Turn trunk to face right leg, pulling right hip back to make hips even. Raise kneecaps, straighten legs.

2. Exhale, bend right knee to form a right angle. Take a few breaths. Keep back erect, left leg straight.

3. Exhale, bend forward from hips. Rest chest on thigh. Take a few breaths.

4. Exhale, shift weight to right foot and lift entire body. Arms, trunk and left leg form a parallel line with floor. Hips and leg are aligned as in Supported Runner's Balance. Hold for a few breaths, release to number 2. Reverse.

Benefits: Tones abdominal muscles, stretches and strengthens legs and improves agility and balance.

23. New Leg Balance

1. Do the Triangle (p.20) to the right.

2. Exhale, bend right knee, place right fingertips on floor about a foot away from right foot. Rest left arm on side.

3. Exhale, straighten right leg, lifting straight left leg. Balance on right fingertips with weight on right leg. Keep left hip and shoulder back, right buttock tucked under, chest expanded.

4. (If you can't keep the right leg straight, place your right palm on a low chair. This exercise can also be done with the back against a wall.) Hold five to ten seconds, bend the right knee, release to Triangle. Reverse.

Benefits: Strengthens ankles, stretches legs and loosens hips.

24. Splits

1. Warm up for Splits by doing the Groin Stretch (p.31). Then do the Groin Stretch between two sturdy chairs, placing your forearms on the chairs.

2. Exhale, using arms for balance, lift hips and straighten front leg.

3. Exhale, carefully slide front heel forward, keeping hips even. Use your arms to keep the weight off your legs. Hold for a few breaths. Change legs.

4. The Splits are a challenge. Eventually you can work without chairs, but the arms should always carry the body's weight until the hips and legs are very flexible.

Benefits: Intense stretch for legs and hips.

1. Ledge Stretch

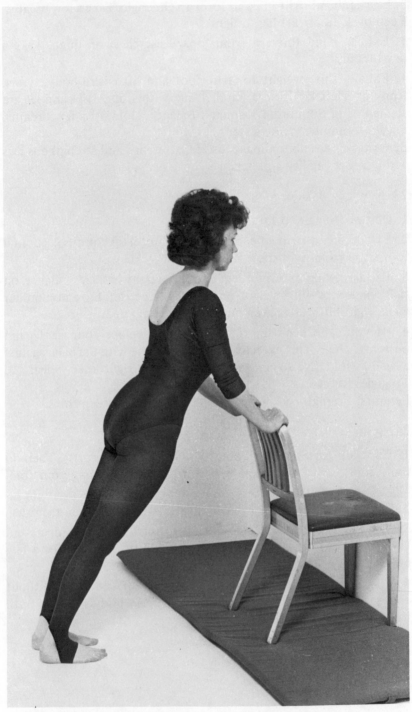

Ledge Stretch benefits the Achilles tendon by stretching it.

1. Ledge Stretch (CONT'D.)

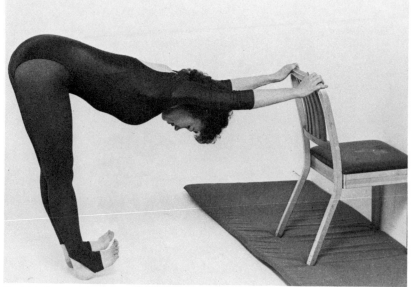

Rock back onto your heels in a smooth movement.

3. Bent Knee Calf Stretch

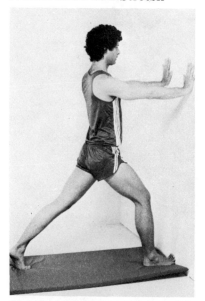

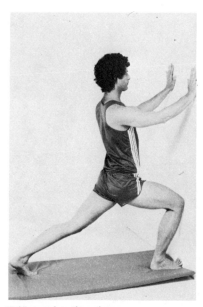

Bend the front knee toward the wall in Bent Knee Calf Stretch.

This stretches the calves.

4. The Wall Chair

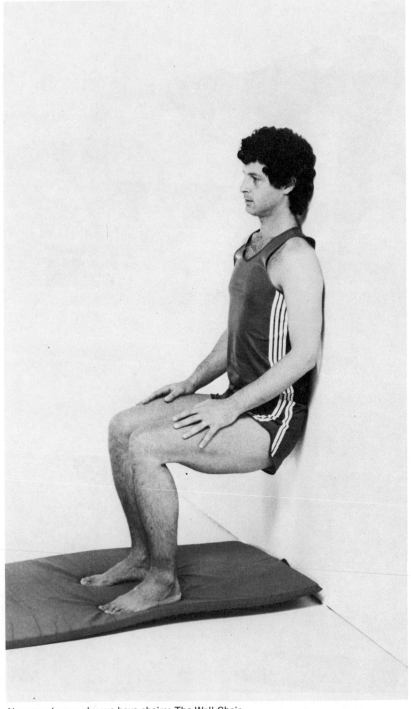

Now you know why we have chairs: The Wall Chair.

5. Invisible Chair

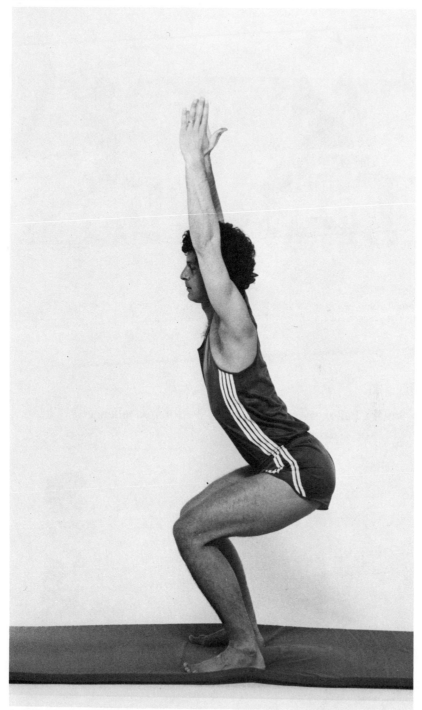

Invisible Chair strengthens quadriceps, improves balance.

6. The Dancer

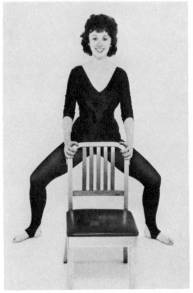

Normally you would use a door jamb to do The Dancer, but a chair will work.

7. Proud Warrior

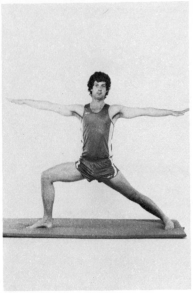

Yes, this is a Proud Warrior.

8. Squat Challenge I

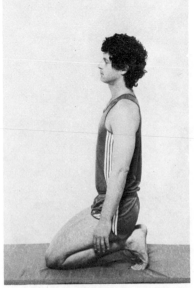

Sit back on your heels in Squat Challenge I.

9. Squat Challenge II

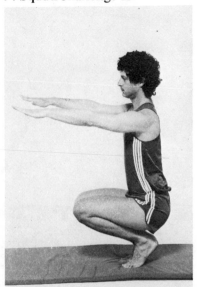

In Squat Challenge II, the arms are held out in front for balance.

10. Squat Challenge III

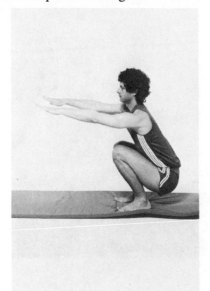

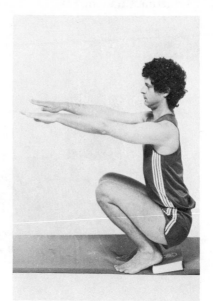

In Squat Challenge III, press your heels to the floor. Use a book under the heels if they don't touch the floor.

The Squat Challenge series is good for stretching the Achilles tendon.

11. Sitting Challenge I

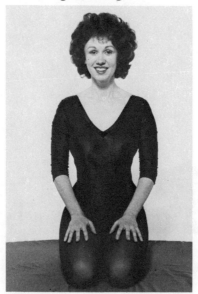

Step 2 position for Sitting Challenge I.

12. Sitting Challenge II

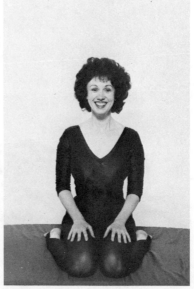

Bring the feet wider apart in Sitting Challenge II, than in Challenge I.

13. Sitting Challenge III

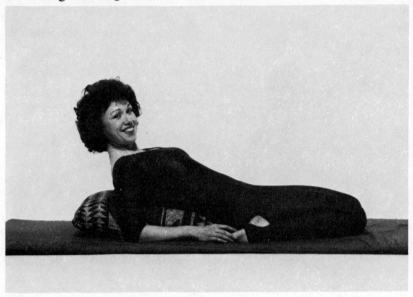

Sitting Challenge III is just that, a challenge.

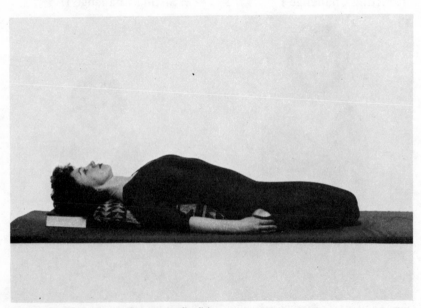

In Challenge III, your thighs must be flexible.

14. Sitting Challenge IV

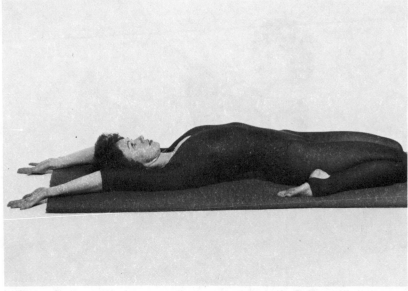

In Sitting Challenge IV, the arms are extended above the head. This is an intense stretch.

15. Sitting Challenge V

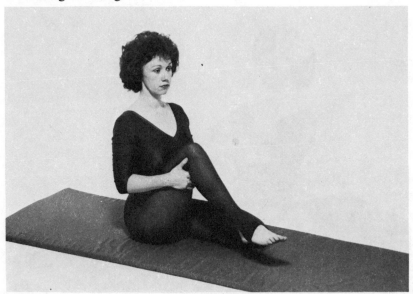

Bring a knee to your chest, supporting back of thigh with a hand in Sitting Challenge V.

(CONT'D NEXT PAGE)

15. Sitting Challenge V (CONT'D.)

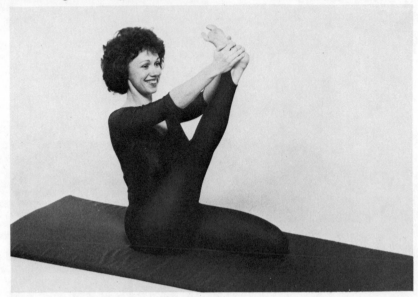

Straighten the bent leg toward ceiling.

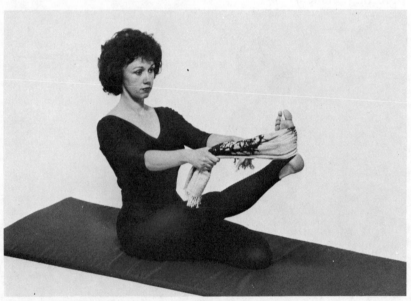

Use a towel if the back rounds.

16. Resting Leg Stretch

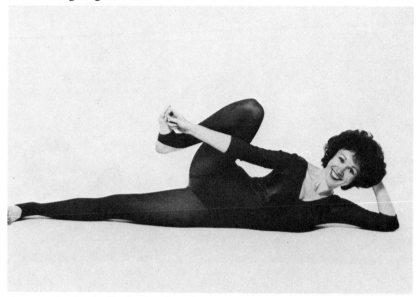

You can relax for the Resting Leg Stretch.

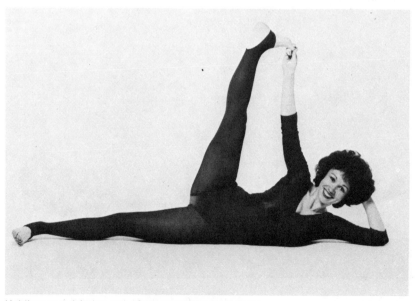

Holding your right leg at the foot, extend leg straight up.

17. Resting Leg Lift I

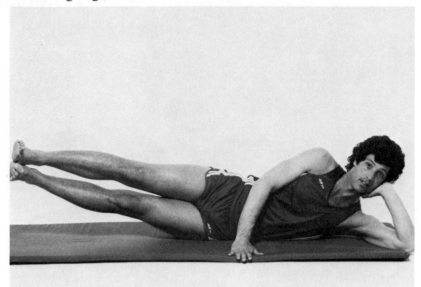

Straighten both legs and lift toward ceiling while resting on your side, in Resting Leg Lift I.

18. Resting Leg Lift II

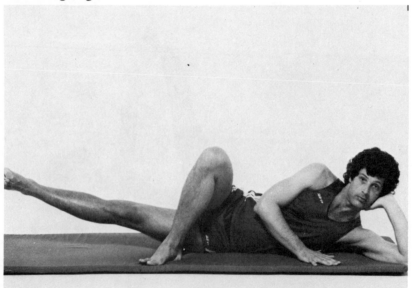

In Resting Leg Lift II, cross one leg over the other and lift straight leg.

19. Archer

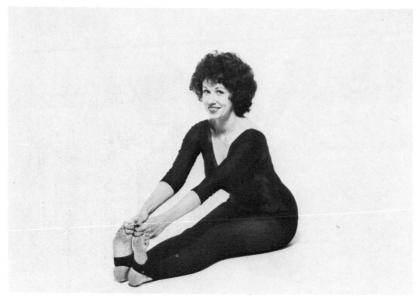

Archer starts out simply enough; touch your toes.

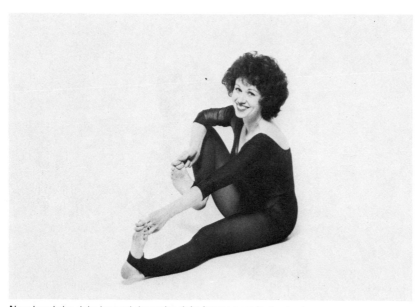

Now bend the right leg and draw the right knee toward your body.

(CONT'D NEXT PAGE)

19. Archer (CONT'D.)

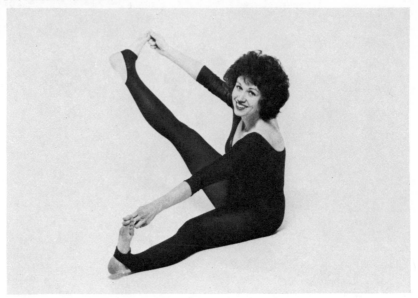

Stretch that right leg out to the side.

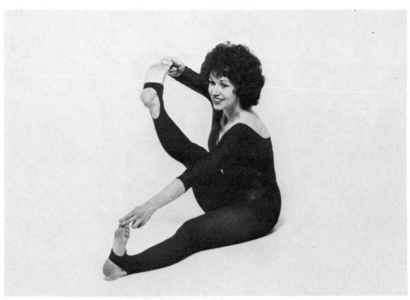

Bring the stretched leg up to your ear.

20. Thigh Stretch

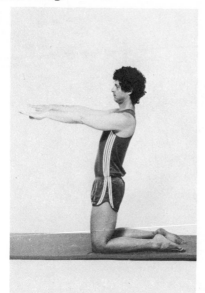

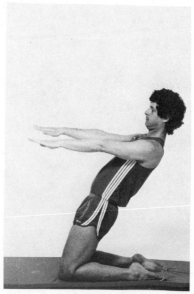

You needn't turn toward Mecca to do Thigh Stretch.

Now lean your entire body back; hold five to ten seconds.

21. Supported Runner's Balance

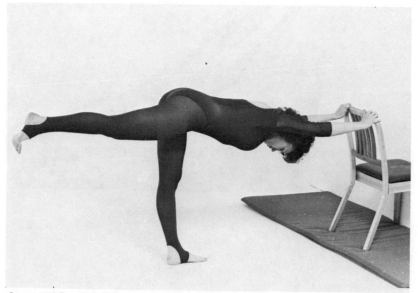

Supported Runner's Balance is similar to Back Extender, but you lift a leg.

22. Runner's Balance

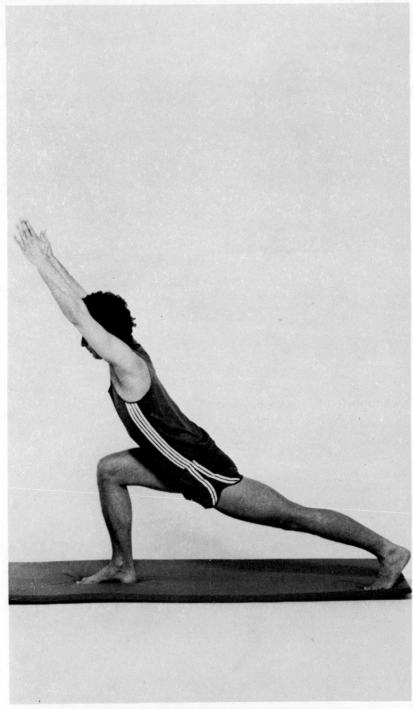

Runner's Balance stretches the Achilles tendon and improves balance.

22. Runner's Balance (CONT'D.)

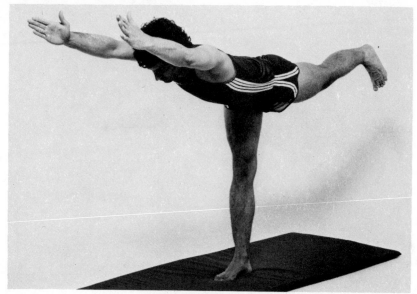

No, it isn't Flying Leap, but Runner's Balance.

23. New Leg Balance

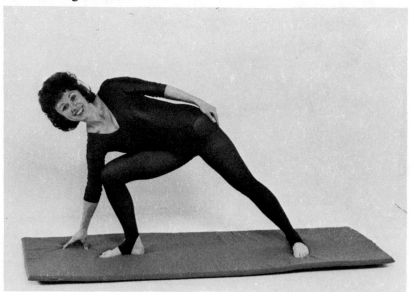

New Leg Balance stretches the leg muscles.

(CONT'D NEXT PAGE)

23. New Leg Balance (CONT'D.)

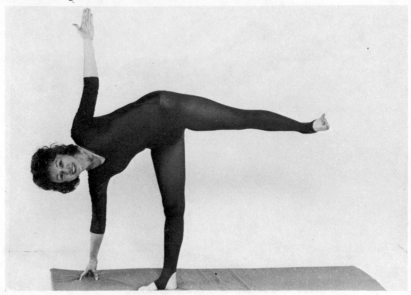

Bring your left leg off the floor.

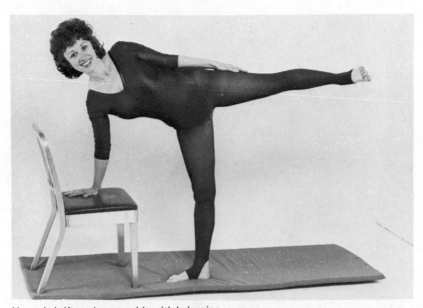

Use a chair if you have trouble with balancing.

(CONT'D.)

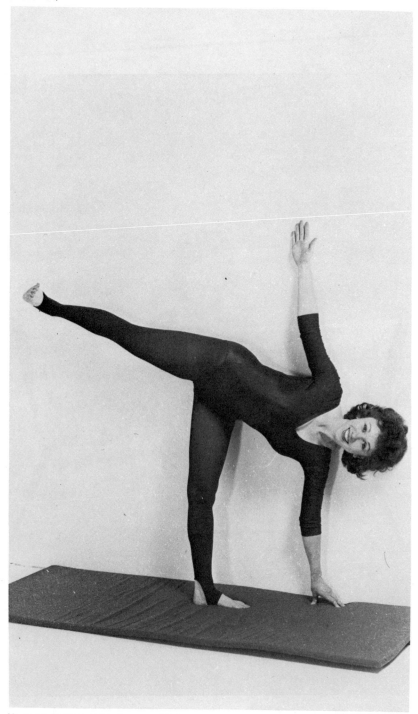

Now reverse pose and balance on left leg.

24. Splits

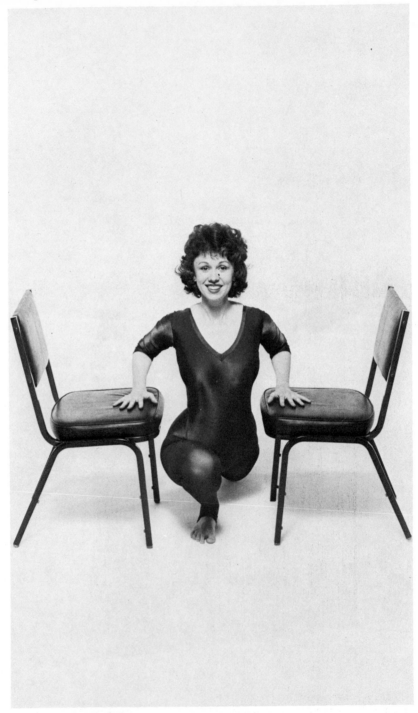

Use two chairs to do Splits.

24. Splits (CONT'D.)

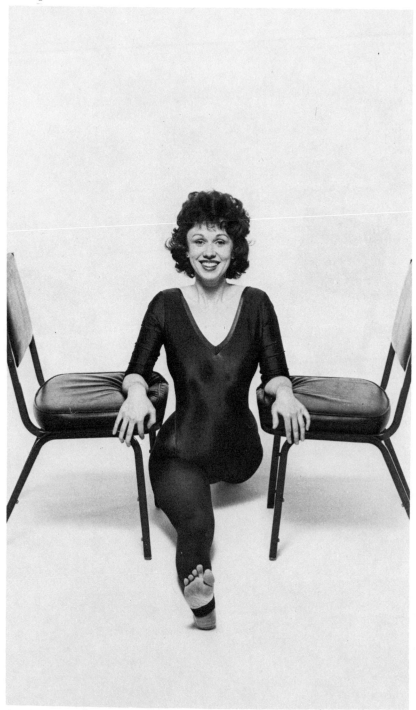

Carefully slide your front heel forward.

(CONT'D NEXT PAGE)

24. Splits (CONT'D.)

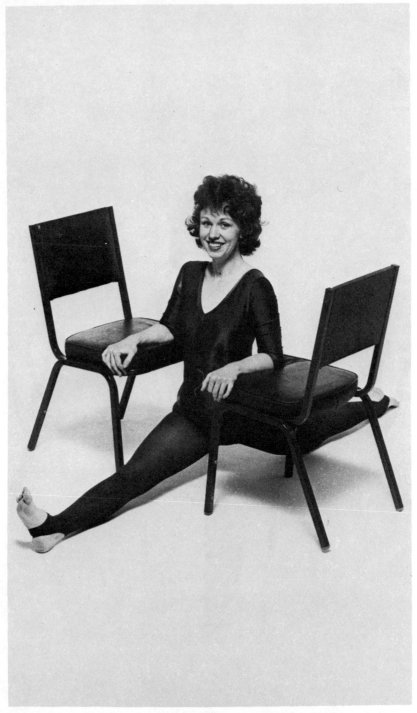

Use the chairs until you develop good flexibility.

6

Hips, Waist and Abdomen

The good news is very good: the muscles of the abdomen and lower back can be strengthened by exercise. The bad news is that they can also remain weak with exercise, and that applies to runners. Running shortens and tightens the muscles of the lower back, resulting in a relatively weak abdominal area. Obviously, the key is to exercise correctly.

"If an athlete has weak abdominals, and tight hip flexors, he or she is headed for lower back pain or injury," according to exercise physiologist Dick Lewis. Dr. Lewis, professor at the University of Arkansas at Little Rock, and a runner for thirty years, teaches his students the importance of maintaining optimum pelvic alignment through stretching. The abdominal muscles that cross the front of the lower torso and the psoas muscle of the back determine the tilt of the pelvis, as do the muscles, ligaments and tendons of the upper leg. If the pelvis tips forward, the result is a swayback, which is characterized by a protruding belly and an overarched lower back. Each running stride contracts the psoas muscle to lift the leg. These repeated contractions of the psoas tend to shorten the muscle, rendering it tight and inflexible. The corresponding abdominals will thus be relatively weakened. This swayback posture can also compress the discs of the lower back, causing lower-back pain.

So in order to exercise the abdominals, the pelvis must be stabilized so that only the abdominal muscles work. In other words, when you exercise, flatten your lower back to flatten your belly! This action is particularly evident in traditional leg lifts: the pelvis should be tilted so that the lower back rests as flat on the floor as possible. If the lower back arches, the psoas—not the abdominals— is lifting the legs. This is a classic example of how exercise done incorrectly simply reinforces a weakness.

The hip joint area can be conditioned to provide more flexibility with exercise. This greater flexibility will insure better, more efficient leg action in running, especially in hill work, and will help prevent painful groin and hip injury. The muscles of the buttocks are large and powerful. Strengthening them and increasing flexibility in the hip joints can add to the strength and stability of your back.

Please take note of the exercise instructions in this chapter. If you're serious about conditioning that which is covered by your running shorts, the time spent reading the instructions will help produce a flatter abdomen, a more taut waistline, a stronger lower back and more flexible hips.

1. Dancer's Stretch I

1. Stand with the feet about 3 - 3½ feet apart. Turn the feet out thirty degrees. Stretch the arms straight up.

2. Exhale, bend from hips to the right. Do not twist the trunk. Press down through the balls of the feet, lift kneecaps. Hold for two breaths. Exhale up. Repeat several times. Change sides.
Benefits: Tones waist, abdomen.

2. Dancer's Stretch II

1. Do Dancer's Stretch I. Hold for two breaths.

2. Exhale, drop left side of body, forming a flat back to the right. Straighten legs and arms and look at the floor. Hold for two breaths.

3. Exhale, push right hip forward, lift left hip, coming back to Dancer's Stretch I. Hold for two breaths, exhale up. Repeat several times, change sides.
Benefits: Loosens hips, elongates back.

3. Dancer's Stretch III

1. Do Dancer II, hold "flat back" to right.

2. Exhale, move slowly from the hips, bring flat back position around to the left. Keep body parallel with the floor during this movement. Legs and arms are straight.

3. Hold flat back to the left for a few breaths. Do Dancer I. Exhale up. Repeat sequence on left side.
Benefits: Tones waist, abdomen, strengthens hips and back.

4. Dancer's Stretch IV

1. Do Dancer II to the right. Hold for two breaths.

2. Exhale, simultaneously relax back, hold elbows and swing down from the hips and back up to left flat back position. Hold for two breaths.

3. Do Dancer I. Exhale up and repeat sequence to the left.
Benefits: Combining I - IV as a long exercise strengthens the legs and arms, brings hip flexibility and tones the waist and abdomen. abdomen.

5. Right Angle

1. Sit on the floor with the legs together and straight, feet and back perpendicular to the floor. Interlock fingers.

2. Exhale, straighten arms along ears, pushing palms toward ceiling. Shoulders stay down, chest expands, back remains erect. Hold five to ten seconds, keeping face and neck relaxed. Repeat, changing interlock of fingers by placing the other thumb on top.
Benefits: Improves posture, slims waist.

6. Sitting Side Stretch

1. Sit erect with the knees bent, left heel in right groin, right heel in front. Place fingers behind ears, lift elbows and breastbone.

2. Exhale, bring right elbow to right knee. Keep left shoulder and elbow back. Hold ten to fifteen seconds. Inhale up.

3. Exhale, bend to right, elbow toward floor. Keep both elbows in line with hips, left thigh and knee down. Hold five to ten seconds. Inhale up. Change sides.
Benefits: Slims waist.

7. Chair Twist I

1. Sit erect, facing sideways in a chair, right side toward chair. Place both hands on chair back.

2. Exhale, simultaneously turn torso to right, bringing right hand to chair seat. Push right hip slightly forward, keep back erect, shoulders down, chest expanded. Neck and face should be relaxed.

Hold five to ten seconds. Reverse.
Benefits: Slims waist, increases spinal flexibility.

8. Chair Twist II

1. Sit erect in chair, feet and knees slightly apart. Stretch arms up along ears.
2. Exhale, turn to right. Place hands on chair back. Push right hip slightly forward, keep feet on floor. Press right elbow into body to expand chest. Hold five to ten seconds. Reverse.
Benefits: Loosens shoulders, expands chest, slims waist.

9. Wall Twist

1. Sit about six to eight inches away from wall in position of Sitting Challenge I (p. 60), with your left side to wall. Shift weight to sit on left hip. Stretch arms up.
2. Exhale, turn to left. Bend elbows, place hands on wall at chest level. Use your arms to help you turn while keeping back erect, shoulders down. Lift and expand chest. Press right buttock down to floor. Hold ten to fifteen seconds. Release and reverse.
Benefits: Slims waist, increases spinal flexibility; good preparation for Yoga Twist.

10. Yoga Twist

1. Sit in position for Sitting Challenge I. Shift weight to left, sit on left hip. Place right hand on left knee, left hand behind left buttock.
2. Exhale, turn to left allowing right hip and buttock to roll forward. Keep the torso perpendicular to floor, resisting the urge to lean in to the left as you turn. Walk left hand around on floor for balance. Press right buttock down when you've turned as far as possible. Neck should remain loose. Hold five to ten seconds. Reverse.
Benefits: Increases flexibility in back, slims waist.

11. Leg Lifts I

1. Lie on back. Stretch arms alongside ears. Bend both knees and place the feet parallel to each other on floor. Press lower back down. Bring left knee to chest.
2. Exhale, straighten left leg, pushing ball of foot toward ceiling. Press down on waist—and not on head—as you lift. Hold ten to fifteen seconds. Repeat several times, change legs. Continue to Leg Lift II.

12. Leg Lift II

1. Lie on back, arms along body, palms down. Place feet together and perpendicular to floor.

2. Exhale, press waist down, lift left leg, keeping both legs straight. Hold ten to fifteen seconds, release and repeat. Change legs. Continue to Leg Lift III.

13. Leg Lift III

1. Lie on back. Place feet together and perpendicular to floor. If lower back is strong, bring arms alongside ears, palms up. If you have a weak back, keep arms by body, palms down.

2. Exhale, press waist to floor and lift legs ninety degrees. Hold for a few breaths. Exhale, lower legs to sixty degrees, hold for two breaths. Exhale, lower legs to thirty degrees, hold for one breath. Exhale, lower to floor. Build to lifting to thirty, sixty, and ninety degrees with longer holds on the way up and down.

Benefits: Leg Lift sequence strengthens the abdomen and back.

14. Belly Twister I

1. Lie on back, arms in "T" position, palms down. Lift knee to chest.

2. Exhale, roll the knees to the floor on the left. Exhale, keeping the legs together, stretch both legs out straight, keeping the feet slightly above the floor. Hold for a few breaths and then bend knees; roll back up to starting position. Change sides.

Benefits: Strengthens abdomen and back.

15. Belly Twister II

1. Lie on back, arms in "T" position, legs straight, feet together.

2. Exhale, lift legs, shift hips to point feet toward left hand.

3. Exhale, lower legs until the feet are near the left hand and about one inch from floor. Keep shoulders and palms on floor. (Holding a piece of sturdy furniture with your right hand will help.) Hold for a few breaths. Exhale, lift legs up and reverse.

Benefits: Excellent strengthener for abdominal muscles.

16. The Boat

1. Sit erect and balance with the knees drawn into the chest, hands under thighs, feet slightly off floor.

2. Exhale, support legs and straighten them, keeping the back erect. Balance for a few breaths and then release hands. Keep arms

straight and parallel with the floor. Hold for a few breaths and release.

Benefits: Stretches and strengthens legs; strengthens abdomen and back.

17. Butterfly

1. Sit with knees bent, feet close to buttocks. Reach between knees and hold big toes.

2. Exhale, straighten legs as you sit erect. Keep feet together, chest expanded, shoulders down. Hold for a few breaths. (If you round your back or bend your knees, try using a belt or tie around the feet. Hold the ends of the tie with both hands. Legs and back can stay straight this way.)

3. Exhale, lift breastbone and separate legs. Take a few breaths, return to number 2. Release.

Benefits: Strengthens abdomen, improves balance, stretches legs.

18. Flat Boat

1. Sit and balance, with knees to chest. Interlock fingers and place hand behind head.

2. Exhale, simultaneously straighten and lower legs and trunk slowly, until both are about thirty degrees from the floor. Expand chest. Take a few breaths, release to floor. Build to ten to fifteen seconds.

Benefits: Excellent for abdomen.

19. Roll Ups

1. Lie on your back. Bend your knees, interlock fingers behind head.

2. Exhale, tuck the chin under and lift head and upper back. Bring the elbows to thighs. Hold for a few breaths. Roll down and repeat. Build to ten to fifteen repetitions.

3. Exhale, come up as in number 2. Take left elbow to right knee, right elbow to left knee. Roll down and repeat.

Benefits: Strengthens abdominals, oblique muscles.

20. The Soft Pretzel

1. Squat with your feet together, heels flat (use a book under your heels if they don't touch the floor.)

2. Exhale, separate knees with chest. Hold heels with hands, rest head on floor. Hold for twenty to thirty seconds.
Benefits: Exercises and strengthens the pelvic area.

21. Indian Cobbler I

1. Sit in Right Angle (p. 87). Bend knees and turn soles of feet together.
2. Exhale, use hands to bring feet closer to groin. Relax inner thighs and allow knees to fall out and down. Keep back straight with chest expanded. Hold twenty to thirty seconds. Build to one minute.
Benefits: Loosens hips.

22. Indian Cobbler II

1. Sit on a small pillow with your back against the wall. Bend knees and do Indian Cobbler I.
2. Inhale, lift chest. Exhale, slide shoulder blades down and flatten them against wall. Relax groin. Use your hands to gently coax thighs down. Hold twenty to thirty seconds.
Benefits: Increases awareness of correct posture in this exercise.

23. Reclining Indian Cobbler (If your back and hips are stiff, try this variation.)

1. Lie on your side with your knees bent, buttocks touching wall.
2. Exhale, roll on your back. Place your feet on the wall, soles touching each other. Use your hands to pull the heels down and to gently press thighs to wall. Slide shoulder blades toward buttocks. Hold for about thirty seconds.
Benefits: Loosens hips without straining back.

24. Hip Opener

1. Lie on back with feet together and perpendicular to floor, palms down.
2. Exhale, lift left leg. Hold the left big toe with left thumb and next two fingers. (Hold lower on leg if this is not possible with a straight leg.)
3. Exhale, keeping right buttock pressed to floor, lower left leg to side. Take a few breaths. Keep right buttock and shoulder down. Exhale back up, repeat. Reverse.
Benefits: Loosens hips, tones legs.

25. Rock-A-Baby I

1. Sit in position of Right Angle (p.87). Bend left leg. Slip right hand under left ankle, left hand under knee.

2. Exhale, lift left leg. Gently twist hands back and forth for fifteen to twenty seconds. Reverse. If this is easy, continue to Rock-A-Baby II.

26. Rock-A-Baby II

1. Sit in position of Rock-A-Baby I. Slip the arch of the left foot into the right elbow, hold the left knee in the left elbow.

2. Exhale, gently twist elbows back and forth for ten to fifteen seconds. Reverse.
Benefits: Loosens hips.

27. Closed Gate

1. Kneel on the floor. Stretch the right leg out to the right, keeping it in line with the left knee. Stretch the arms out horizontally.

2. Exhale, bend from the hips to the right. Press the right foot down and bring the left arm over the left ear. Right hand rests on right straight leg. Roll the left hip and shoulder back, push the right buttock forward. Hold ten to fifteen seconds. Reverse.
Benefits: Stretches legs, tones abdomen and loosens hips.

28. Backward Groin Stretch

1. Sit in position of Sitting Challenge I (p.60). Gently reach back and place hands on floor, fingers pointing toward knees, fingertips in line with toes.

2. Exhale, squeeze buttocks, tuck tail under and lift. Straighten arms, and hold body like a slant board. Hang head loosely. (This exercise should be avoided if you have a neck injury.) Hold ten to fifteen seconds.
Benefits: Stretches groin, strengthens buttocks and back.

29. Standing Bow

1. Do Growing Taller (p.16) about an arm's length from a sturdy table. Bend left leg, hold left ankle with left hand. Stretch right arm to front, palm down.

2. Exhale, lean forward, stretch right arm on table, bringing body horizontal. Lift right kneecap. Lift left foot, keeping left hip level

with right hip. Hold ten to fifteen seconds. Reverse. Eventually you might try doing this exercise without using a table, for a real challenge.

30. The Tree

1. Stand in position of Growing Taller.

2. Exhale, use the right hand to bring right foot high on left inner thigh. Point right toes down. Raise left kneecap. Tuck the tail under and keep the hips level. (Don't allow the right buttock to roll back.) Stretch arms out sideways for balance. Hold for a few breaths. Reverse.

3. As in all balancing exercises, this can be done by using a wall for support and "confidence." Stand with your back close to a wall. Do The Tree, stretch arms up or out to the side.

Benefits: Brings hip flexibility, strengthens legs and improves balance.

1. Dancer's Stretch I

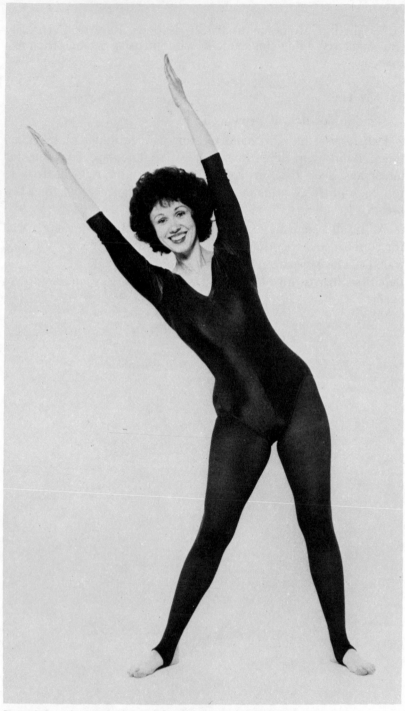

Dancer's Stretch I is a good stretch for the waist and abdomen.

2. Dancer's Stretch II

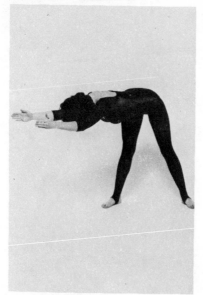

In Dancer's Stretch II, you bend at the waist, arms extended.

3. Dancer's Stretch III

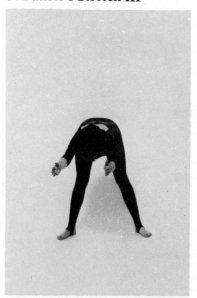

Start by holding "flat back" to right in Dancer's Stretch III.

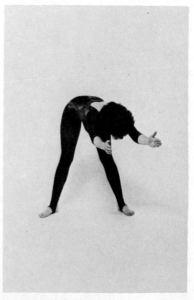

Move slowly from the hips and bring flat back around to the left.

(CONT'D NEXT PAGE)

3. Dancer's Stretch III (CONT'D.)

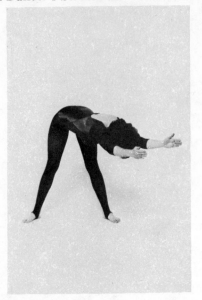

Tones waist and abdomen, and strengthens hips and back.

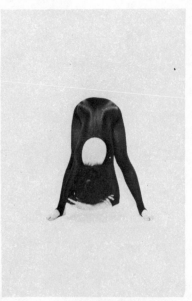

Hold your arms over your head.

4. Dancer's Stretch IV

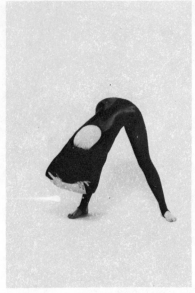

In Dancer's Stretch IV, bend at the waist and swing to the left and right.

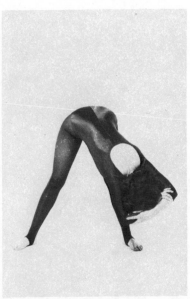

This exercise strengthens the legs and arms.

5. Right Angle

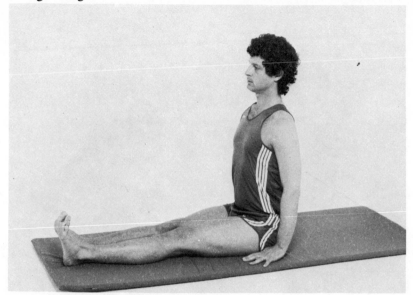

Form a right angle in Right Angle.

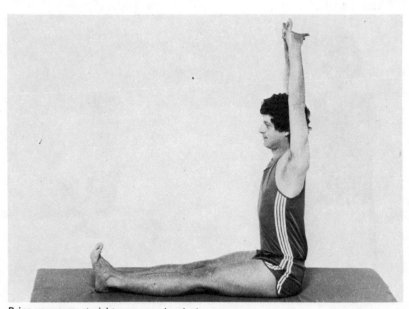

Bring your arms straight over your head, along your ears.

6. Sitting Side Stretch

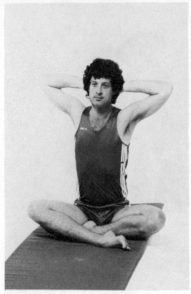

Sitting Side Stretch slims the waist.

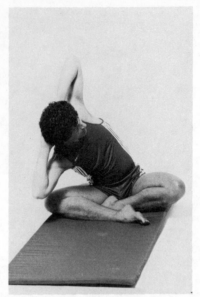

Bring your right elbow to your right knee in this stretch.

7. Chair Twist I

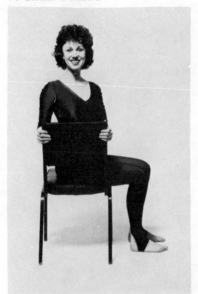

In Chair Twist I, hold onto chair and twist at the waist.

8. Chair Twist II

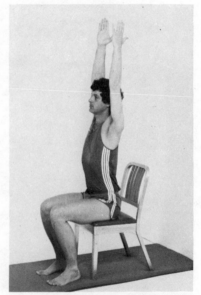

Stretch arms up to begin Chair Twist II.

(CONT'D)

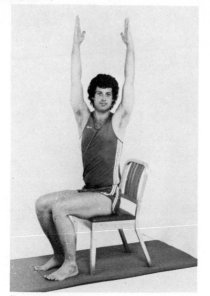

Turn to the right.

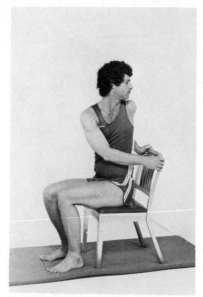

Now hold chair and push your right hip forward.

9. Wall Twist

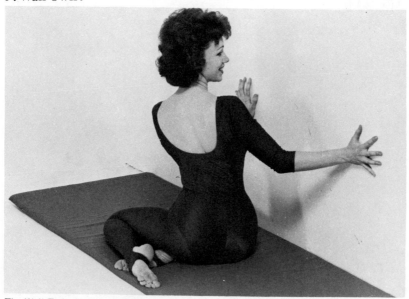

The Wall Twist improves spinal flexibility.

10. Yoga Twist

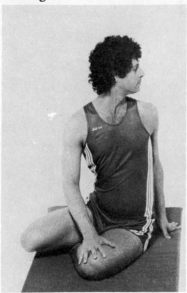

Yoga Twist increases flexibility in the
back and slims the waist.

11. Leg Lift I

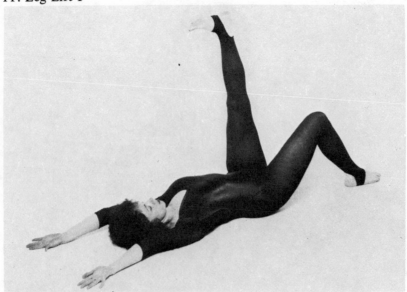

In Leg Lift I you are assured of keeping your back flat because legs are bent at the
knees.

12. Leg Lift II

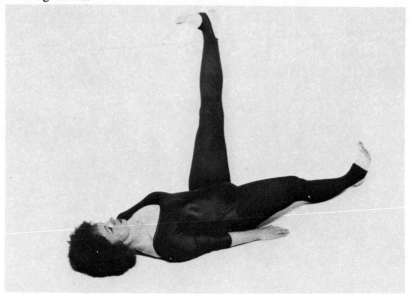

In Leg Lift II, lift a leg to vertical, bring down, then lift other leg.

13. Leg Lift III

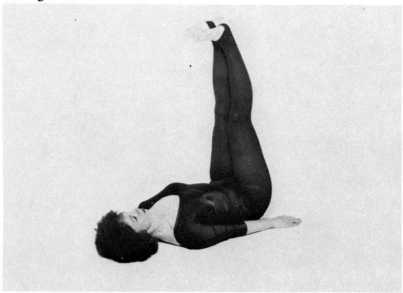

In Leg Lift III, begin with legs vertical, back flat on floor.

(CONT'D.)

13. Leg Lift III (CONT'D.)

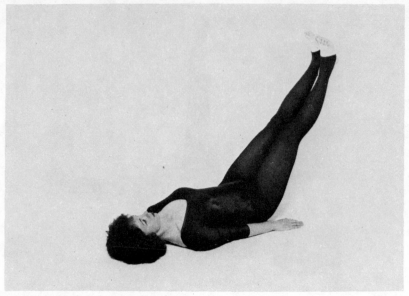

Bring legs, together, down to sixty degrees.

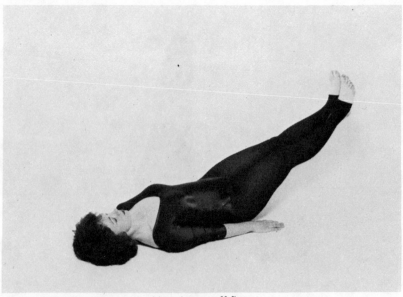

The toughest hold: bring legs to thirty degrees off floor.

14. Belly Twister I

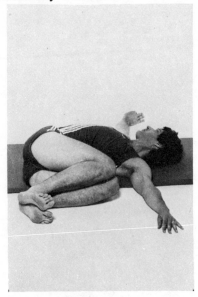

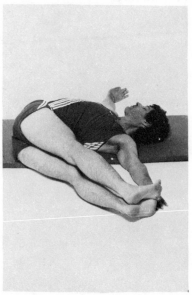

For Belly Twister I, the legs are bent at the knee.

Now extend the legs while you are still bent at the hips.

15. Belly Twister II

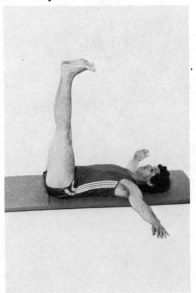

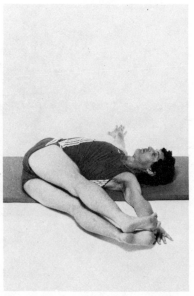

Step I of Belly Twister II is easy enough.

Now lower your legs to the left, keeping them together.

16. The Boat

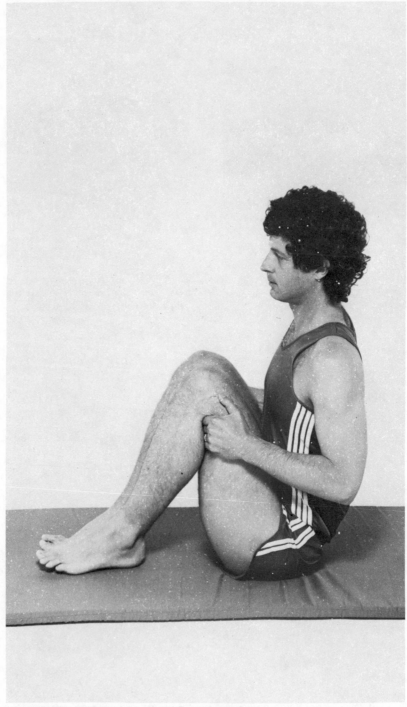

Launch The Boat with knees bent, resting on buttocks.

16. The Boat (CONT'D.)

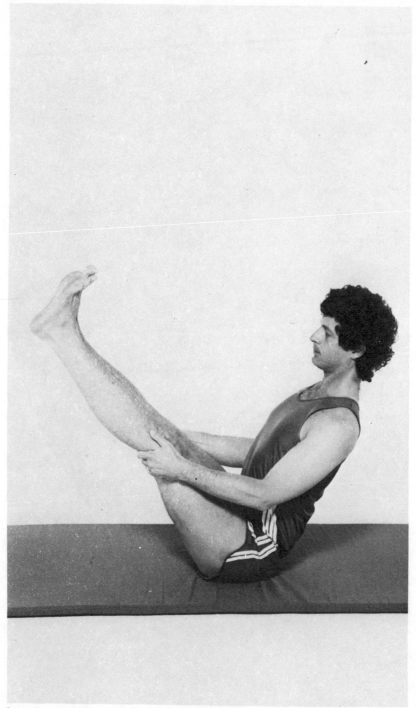

Stay afloat by balancing on buttocks, legs extended.

(CONT'D NEXT PAGE)

16. The Boat (CONT'D.)

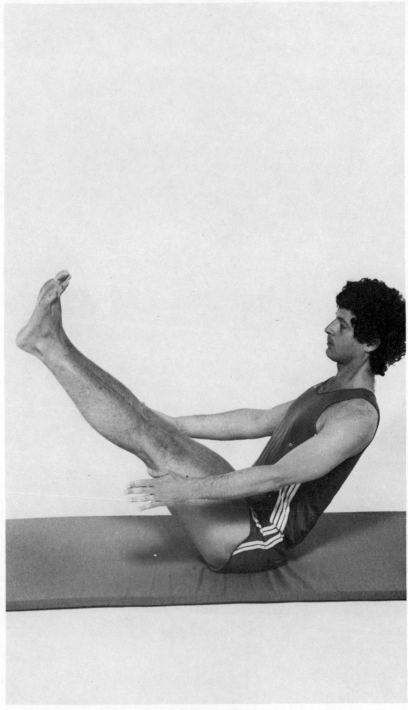

Now release hands from legs and extend them to sides.

17. Butterfly

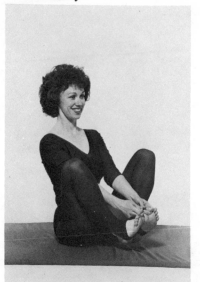

Sit with knees bent to begin Butterfly.

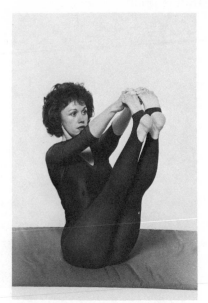

Straighten your legs now, holding your feet with your hands.

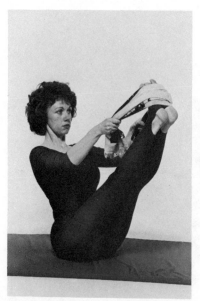

To make it easier, use a towel or tie.

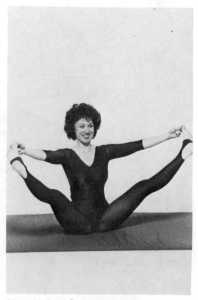

Now do Step 3; separate legs.

18. Flat Boat

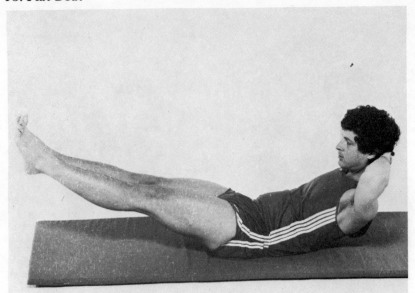

Flat Boat is an excellent conditioner for the abdomen.

19. Roll Ups

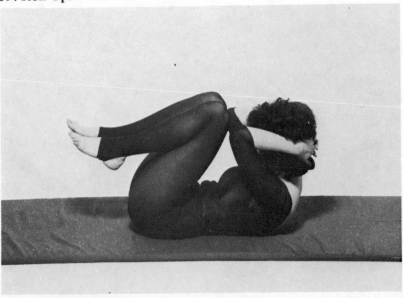

Keep back flat in Roll Ups.

19. Roll Ups (CONT'D.)

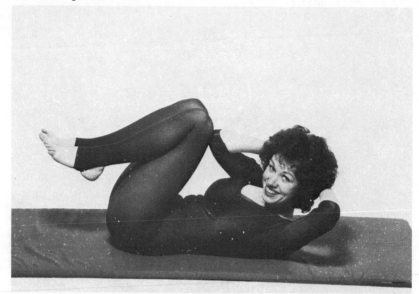

Roll Ups works the abdominals and obliques.

20. Soft Pretzel

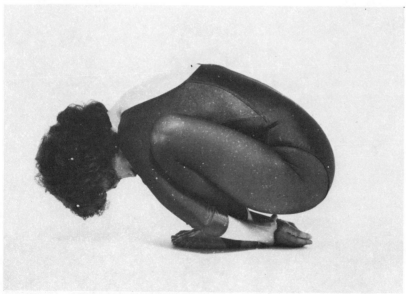

The Soft Pretzel strengthens the pelvic area.

21. Indian Cobbler I

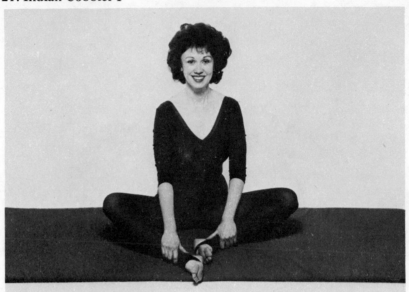

Bring soles of feet together to begin Indian Cobbler I.

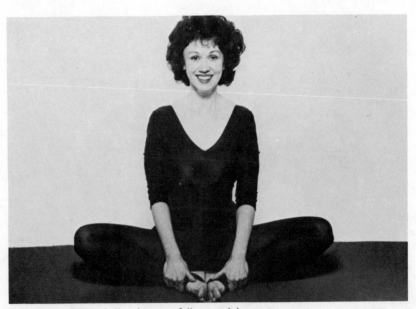

Relax inner thighs and allow knees to fall out and down.

22. Indian Cobbler II

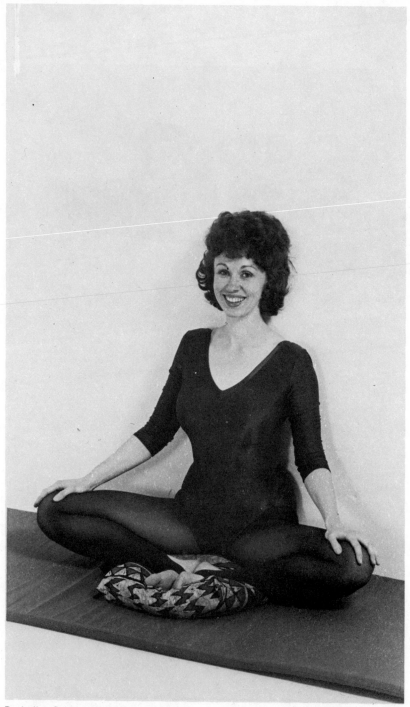

Do Indian Cobbler II with back to a wall.

23. Reclining Indian Cobbler

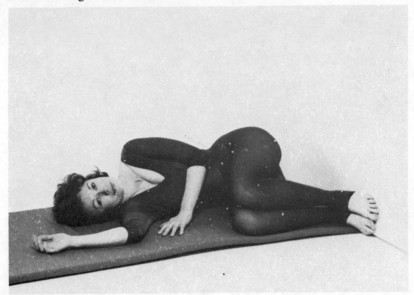

Reclining Indian Cobbler is great for those with stiff hips and backs.

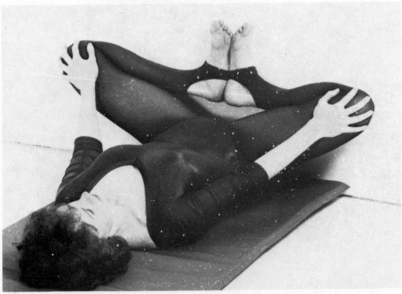

This position calls for resting feet on wall and bringing them toward the floor, stretching groin.

24. Hip Opener

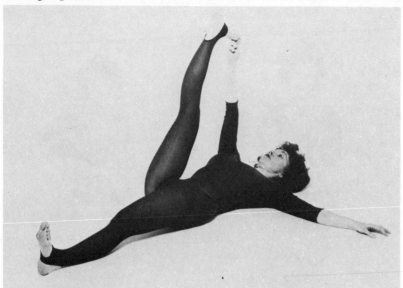

In Hip Opener, if you can't keep leg straight while holding your big toe, bring your hand down the leg.

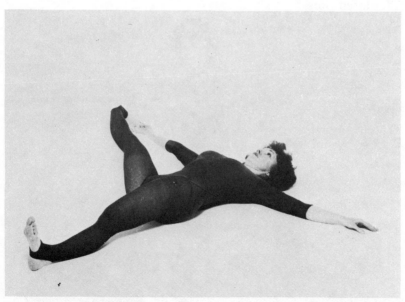

Lower left leg to your left side.

25. Rock A Baby I

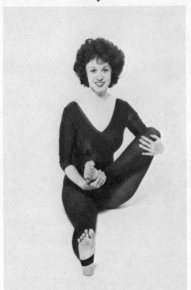

Rock-A-Baby I calls for holding the leg at the knee and ankle. Then twist your hands.

26. Rock A Baby II

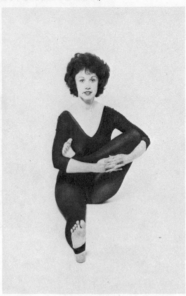

Cradle a leg in Rock-A-Baby II, and then rock your elbows.

27. Closed Gate

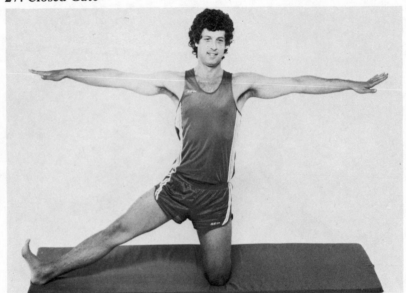

Kneel on your left knee to begin Closed Gate.

27. Closed Gate (CONT'D.)

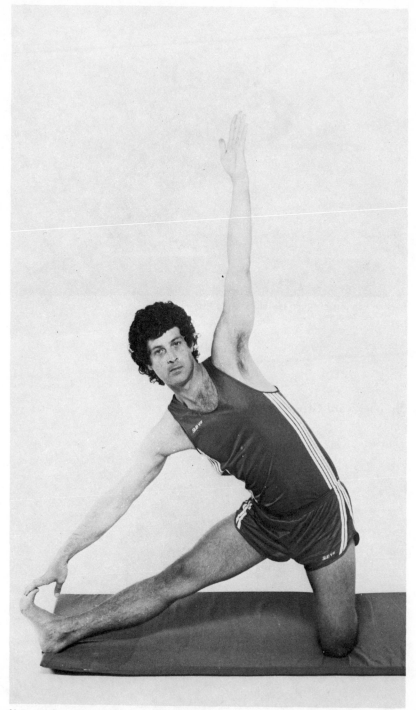

Now touch extended right leg with right hand.

(CONT'D NEXT PAGE)

27. Closed Gate (CONT'D.)

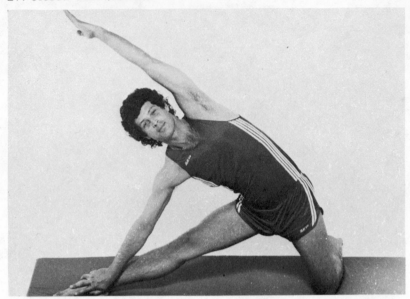

Finally, lean into the right leg. Hold ten to fifteen seconds.

28. Backward Groin Stretch

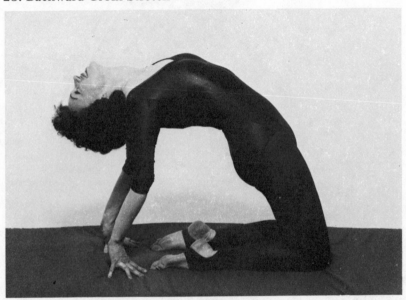

Backward Groin Stretch works the groin and strengthens the buttocks and back.

29. Standing Bow

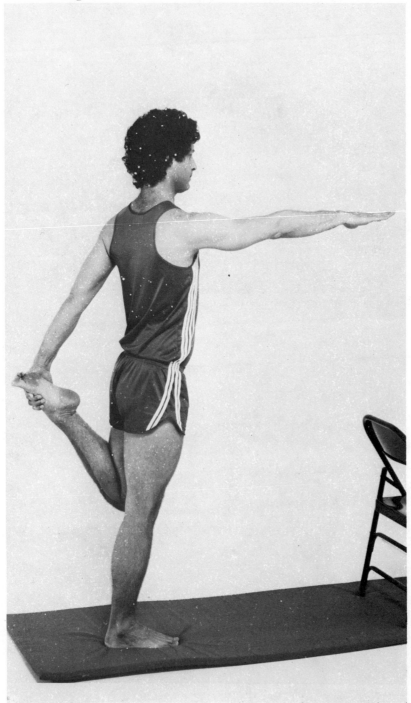

Standing Bow requires considerable balance.

(CONT'D NEXT PAGE)

29. Standing Bow   (CONT'D.)

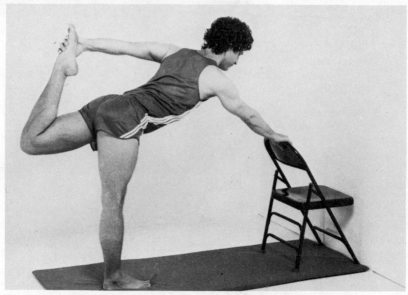

Use a chair or table edge if you have trouble balancing.

30. Tree

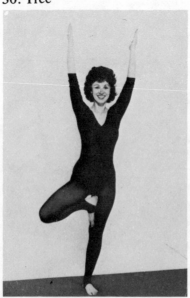

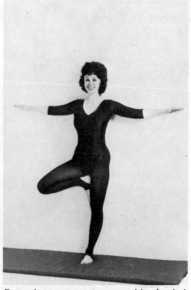

Use your hand, in The Tree, to get your foot onto your inner thigh.

Extend your arms to your sides for balance.

7

Shoulders, Arms and Chest

If we ran on our hands, we'd probably care a lot more about upper body strength. The full potential of our arms, shoulders and chest would be realized. Although most of us will forever run with our feet and legs, that doesn't mean our upper body should just go along totally unprepared for the ride.

The muscles of the upper chest and back give you an amazingly versatile range of movement through the shoulders and arms. When these muscles are inflexible or weak, tension and pain may result, and breathing can be inhibited. This is what causes a postural deviation commonly called "round shoulders." The muscles holding the shoulder blades against the upper posterior thoracic wall lose their tone and the chest collapses. Often, in this condition the upper spine and shoulders seemingly solidify.

The importance of developing strong arms and an expansive chest complemented by flexible shoulders is often ignored by the runner. That's why so many runners suffer from "upper body syndrome." The upper body seems disproportionately small and insignificant, almost child-like. The chest is sagging and narrow. (Sometimes this flattening of the chest is further aggravated by an unbalanced exercise program that focuses solely on taut abdominals.) The shoulders are usually stooped or rounded, and the head may protrude. The arms' musculature seem nonexistent in comparison to the powerful legs.

Specific exercises for this area can increase shoulder flexibility and strengthen the chest, upper back and arms. A sagging chest and inflexible shoulders are not helping your running. In fact, in addition to the overall improved body appearance that these exercises can bring, you may find that an expanded chest gives you better breathing capacity during training. So don't allow the upper body to continue its life as a dullard. It's time for your chest to lift up instead of sagging, and for your shoulders, arms and upper back to strengthen and become more flexible. Allow your top half to contribute to your total athletic performance.

1. Arm Rotations

1. Stand in position of Growing Taller with your feet slightly apart. Stretch the arms out horizontally.
2. Exhale, begin making small clockwise circles with your straight arms, gradually increasing the size of the circle. Do ten repetitions. Reverse. Keep tail tucked under, buttocks firm, legs straight, chest high.
Benefits: Strengthens upper arms and loosens shoulders.

2. Elbow-Arm Chest Stretch

1. Stand in Growing Taller, feet slightly apart. Interlock fingers behind your back. Move both hands to the left by bending the elbows.
2. Exhale, shoulders down, shoulder blades together. Left elbow moves in. Lift the chest on each inhalation. Hold ten to fifteen seconds. Reverse.
Benefits: Expands chest, gives flexibility to shoulders.

3. Chest Expander I

1. Stand in position of Growing Taller, feet slightly apart. Hold a towel between your hands, stretch arms down.
2. Inhale, lift chest. Exhale, squeeze shoulder blades.
3. Exhale, lift arms back, maintaining shoulder blade squeeze. Keep face and neck relaxed. Eventually work without a towel and with interlocked fingers. Hold for a few breaths, release. Repeat.
Benefits: Expands chest and loosens shoulders.

4. Chest Expander II

1. Stand in Growing Taller, feet slightly apart. Interlock fingers behind you or hold a towel. Do Chest Expander I.
2. Exhale, bend forward from the hips, bringing arms up and over. Hold for ten to fifteen seconds with straight legs. Let your upper

arms and chest bring you up.
Benefits: Increases mobility in shoulder girdle.

5. Wall Chest Opener

1. Stand an arm's length from wall, feet parallel and slightly apart. Place your hands on wall at eye-level, shoulder-width apart, fingers pointing up.
2. Exhale, press hands against wall, straighten arms and walk back until your legs are perpendicular and arms fully extended. Do not move hands. Lift tailbone. Keep legs straight. Hold for a few breaths.
Benefits: Increases flexibility in shoulders and legs.

6. Table Hang

1. Put some padding on a sturdy table placed beside a wall. Lie on your back with just your head falling back with gravity. Bend knees and place feet on wall. Close mouth, open eyes.
2. Exhale, take arms back, interlock fingers. Stay for about ten to fifteen seconds. Release arms, take a few breaths, roll over to side to come up.
Benefits: Expands chest.

7. Blanket Roll

1. Roll a blanket into about a three-inch roll. Lie down with blanket under the shoulder blades. Head should rest comfortably on floor. Use a pillow if you feel any neck strain.
2. Exhale, stretch arms back along ears. Push feet away, lower waist to floor. Continue stretching in this way for several breaths. Release, relax the back, and repeat.
Benefits: Expands chest, loosens shoulders.

8. Hands On Your Back

1. Stand in Growing Taller, or sit in position of Sitting Challenge I, or in a chair. Stretch arms up along ears.
2. Exhale, bend right arm, place back of hand on spine, moving right shoulder down. Exhale, bring left hand down to clasp right hand. (Use a towel between the hands if they don't meet.) Keep back erect.
3. Inhale, lift chest. Exhale, bring left elbow closer to ear. Don't turn shoulders to the right. Hold for a few breaths. Reverse.
Benefits: Increases shoulder girdle mobility.

9. Intense Front Stretch I

1. Sit to the front of a sturdy low bench approximately one and a half feet high. Stretch the legs out, feet together. Walk hands back under shoulders. Point fingers toward feet.

2. Exhale, press down on palms and feet, straighten arms, look up. Buttocks are supported by bench. Keep legs straight. Don't over-arch the lower back. Hold for ten to fifteen seconds.
Benefits: Expands chest, strengthens arms and shoulders.

10. Intense Front Stretch II

1. Sit in position of Right Angle (p. 87) with feet two to three inches apart. Place hands behind buttocks, fingers pointing toward the feet.

2. Exhale, straighten arms, press down on balls of feet. Keep the tail tucked under, buttocks firm. Drop head back easily. Hold for a few breaths, release. (If the legs don't remain straight, do this with your toes pushing against a wall.)
Benefits: Stretches the entire front of body.

11. Bridge

1. Lie on your back, knees bent, with the feet parallel and near buttocks. Align feet with the hips. Place arms along body, palms down. Flatten lower back to floor.

2. Exhale, squeeze buttocks, tuck tail under and beginning with the pelvis, slowly lift the back off the floor. Press down through arms, keep buttocks firm, and don't allow the knees or feet to turn out.

3. Hold for a few breaths. Lift buttocks higher, then release by keeping pelvis up as you first lower upper back, then mid and lower back, and finally, the pelvis. Repeat, but this time interlock fingers on floor with straight arms.
Benefits: Increases flexibility in spine and shoulders. Strengthens legs.

12. The High Bridge

When you have mastered the Bridge, try this.

1. Lie on a padded surface in front of a sturdy chair or bench that is against a wall. With knees bent, place your feet on the edge of the chair seat. Feet are slightly apart and parallel. Press lower back down. Place arms along body, palms down.

2. Exhale, do the Bridge (p.122), interlocking fingers and straightening arms under you. Keep knees moving in and feet parallel. Buttocks are firm. Hold for a few breaths, roll down as in the Bridge. Note: If the neck is strained, try placing a mat as in Shoulder Stand.

Benefits: Increases flexibility in spine, expands chest.

1. Arm Rotations

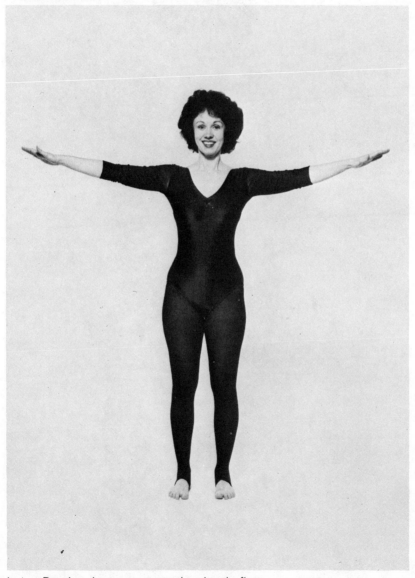

In Arm Rotations, be sure you are anchored to the floor.

2. Elbow-Arm Chest Stretch

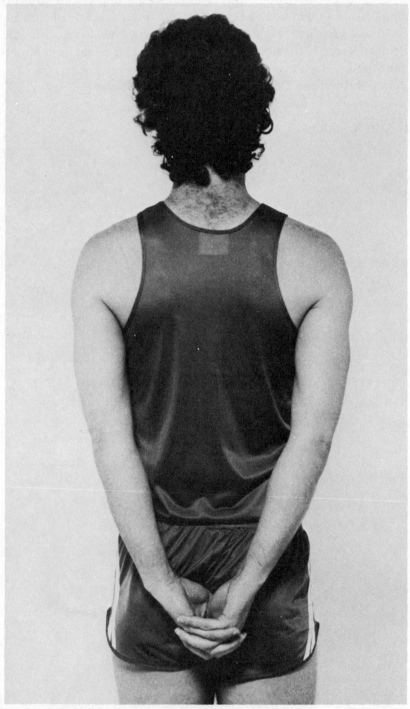

Inhale with arms behind back in Elbow-Arm Chest Stretch.

(CONT'D.)

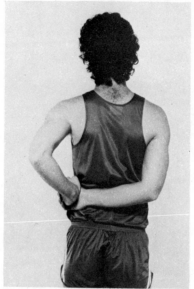 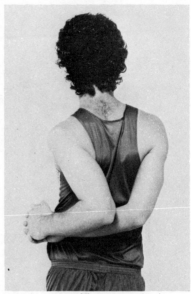

To work shoulder blades, pull one arm behind the back.

Hold for ten to fifteen seconds, then reverse.

3. Chest Expander I

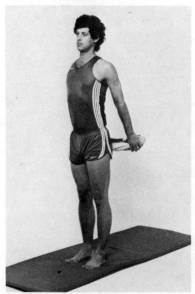 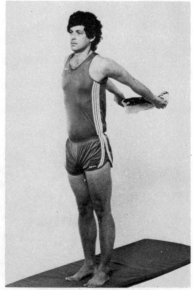

Use a towel for Chest Expander I, to begin.

Lift the towel as high behind your back as you can.

4. Chest Expander II

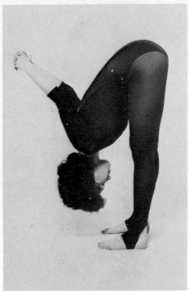

Chest Expander II increases mobility in the shoulder girdle.

5. Wall Chest Opener

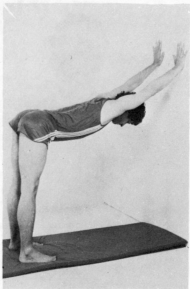

In Wall Chest Opener, walk back from wall until legs are perpendicular and arms are fully extended.

6. Table Hang

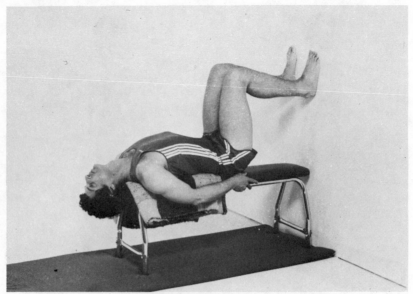

In Table Hang, extend the arms and lean head back.

(CONT'D.)

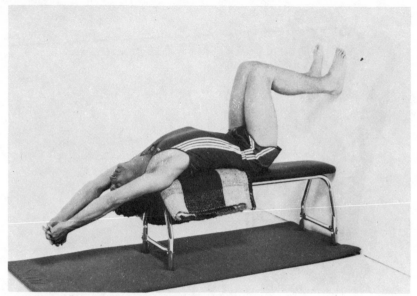

Hold this pose for about ten to fifteen seconds.

7. Blanket Roll

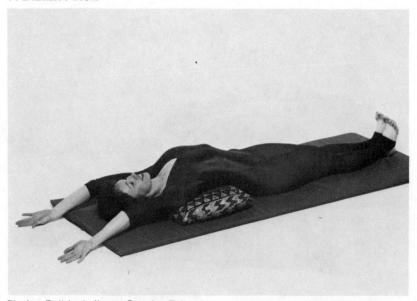

Blanket Roll is similar to Growing Taller, but you are lying on a rolled up blanket.

8. Hands On Your Back

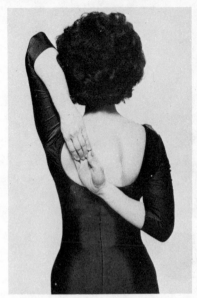

Bend right arm and place back of hand on spine in Hands On Your Back.

9. Intense Front Stretch I

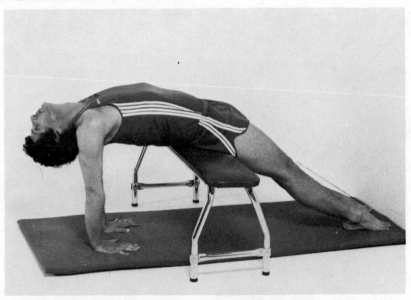

Intense Front Stretch I expands the chest and strengthens arms and shoulders.

11. Bridge

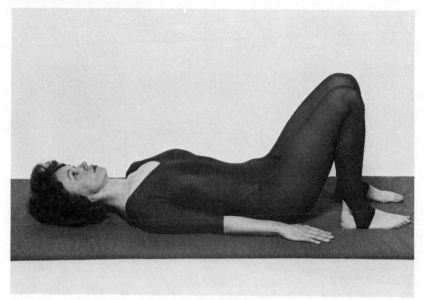

Bridge increases flexibility in the spine and shoulders.

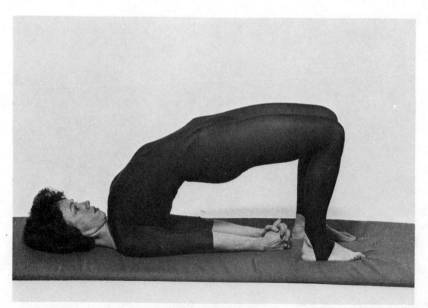

Lift your buttocks off the floor, keeping the shoulders flat.

12. High Bridge

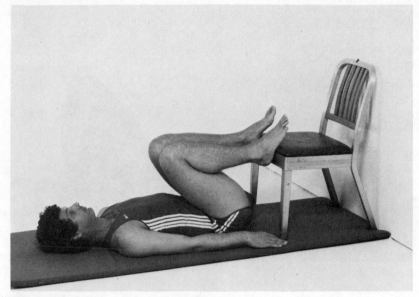

Place a chair against a wall to do High Bridge.

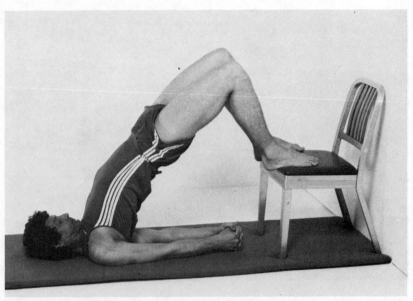

Don't attempt this exercise if you have neck problems.

13. Camel

1. Kneel on a padded surface, knees slightly apart, lower legs and feet parallel. Squeeze buttocks and tuck tail under. Place fists on buttocks and push them forward. (Don't attempt the rest of the exercise if you have neck problems.)

2. Exhale, keep buttocks firm and reach fingers back to soles of feet. Hang head loosely. Turn palms toward thighs. Hold for a few breaths. Build to fifteen to twenty seconds with palms flat on feet.
Benefits: Expands chest, stretches groin and shoulders.

14. Shoulder Squeeze

1. Stand in a doorway. Lean over, round the back, tuck the chin, and carefully place shoulder blades on either side of doorjamb. Keep legs straight, feet parallel.

2. Exhale, lift arms back and up. Press back (not neck) against door. Hold door with hands, if possible. Keep abdomen relaxed. Take a few breaths. Turn feet away from doorjamb and come up. (This exercise can be slightly disorienting at first, so practice with a friend who can guide you.)
Benefits: Increases shoulder mobility, tests back and hamstring flexibility.

15. One Arm Balance

1. Do Downward Dog (p.31) with your heels against a wall.

2. Exhale, roll over to your right side and balance on the right hand and foot. Press the left foot and inner side of the right foot against wall. Left leg rests on right leg. Left arm rests on side. Tuck tail under. Hold for a few breaths with body straight, roll back over to position of Downward Dog. Reverse.
Benefits: Strengthens wrists and arms.

16. Bent Knee Push-Ups

1. Get on all fours, place hands shoulder-width apart in front of the shoulders. Place knees under hips. Tuck tail under.

2. Exhale, bend elbows, lift feet toward buttocks and touch chest to floor. Keep elbows in and tail tucked under, buttocks firm. Inhale up. Repeat five to ten times.
Benefits: Strengthens arms and abdomen.

17. Bench Push-Ups

1. Kneel arm's length away in front of a sturdy bench or chair placed against a wall. Place hands on chair, midfingers parallel and pointing away from you.

2. Exhale, bend elbows and bring chest to chair, straighten legs and tuck tail under. Keep elbows near body. Take a breath.

3. Exhale, straighten arms. Tail is tucked under, body straight. Take a breath.

4. Exhale down. Repeat five to ten times.

Benefits: Strengthens wrists, arms, shoulders and abdomen.

18. Push-Ups

1. Lie on your abdomen. Bend elbows, place hands in front of, or under shoulders. Tuck toes and tail under. Legs straight, feet apart. Inhale while straightening arms and pushing body from floor.

2. Exhale, bend elbows, touch chest to floor. Keep body straight, buttocks firm, tail tucked, elbows in. Inhale up. Repeat as possible. (Moving the hands out from the shoulders works the pectoral muscles of the chest.)

Benefits: Strengthens wrists, arms, shoulders, abdomen.

19. Yoga Arm Balance

1. Sit in position of Right Angle and warm up the hips by doing Rock-A-Baby I or II.

2. Exhale, bend the right leg, hold it at the ankle with the right hand. Lift the leg so that it rests on the upper right arm. Place palms on the floor.

3. Exhale, press down on arms and lift body. Left leg is straight and parallel to floor. Hold for a few breaths. Reverse.

Benefits: Strengthens arms, challenges hip mobility.

13. Camel

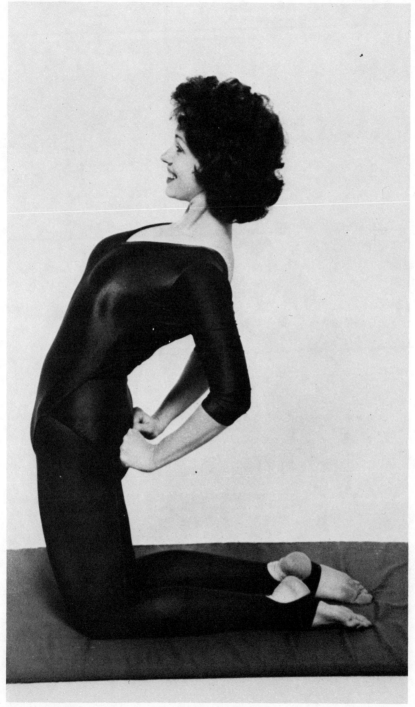

This part of Camel is okay to do if you have neck problems.

(CONT'D NEXT PAGE)

13. Camel (CONT'D.)

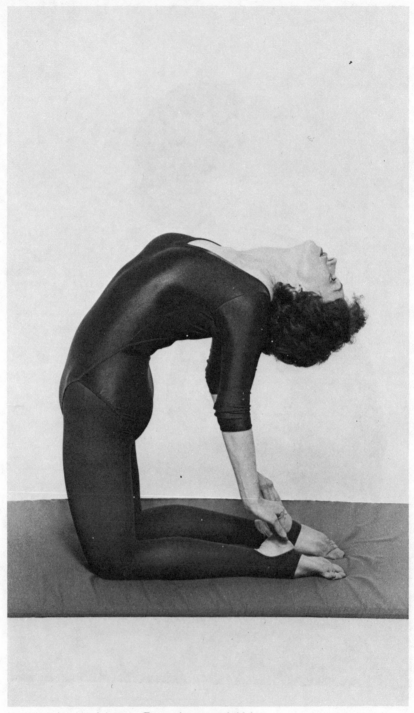

Hang your head back loosely. Turn palms toward thighs.

14. Shoulder Squeeze

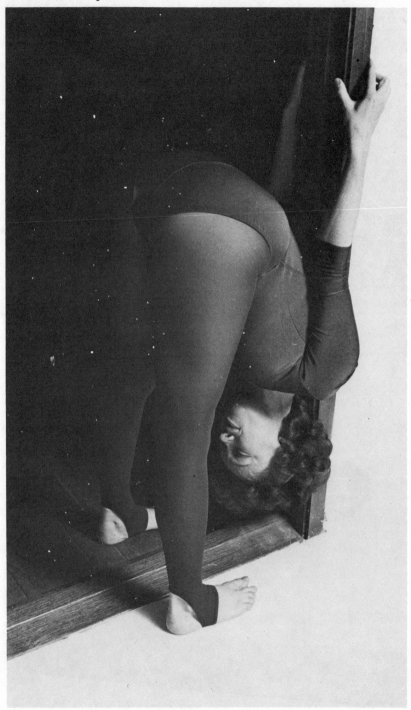

Shoulder Squeeze increases shoulder mobility.

15. One Arm Balance

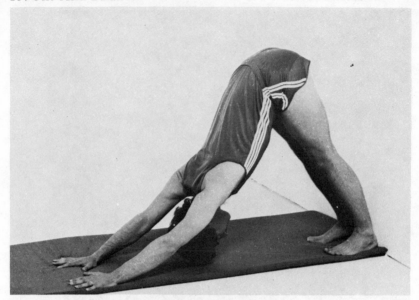

Start One Arm Balance with Downward Dog position.

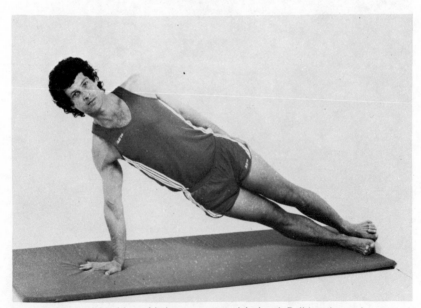

Turn onto your right side and balance on your right hand. Builds wrists and arms.

16. Bent Knee Push-Ups

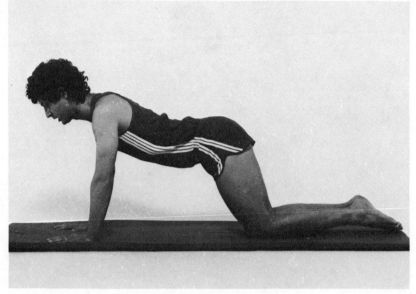

Bent Knee Push-Ups are recommended for those with weak arms.

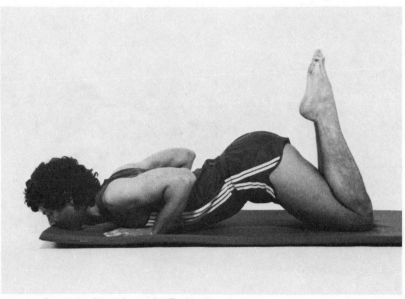

Lift your feet toward your buttocks. Tuck tail.

17. Bench Push-Ups

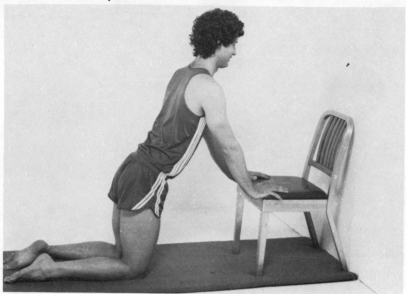

Kneel in front of a chair against a wall in Bench Push-Ups.

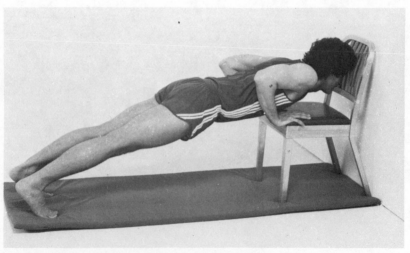

Then extend legs, resting arms on chair in push-up pose.

17. Bench Push-Ups (CONT'D.)

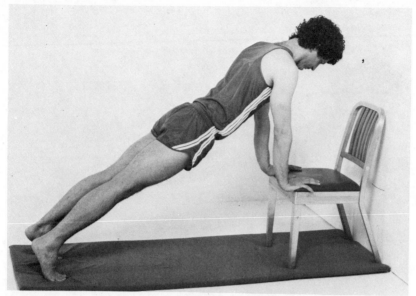

Now do a push-up. Strengthens arms, shoulders and abdomen.

18. Push-Ups

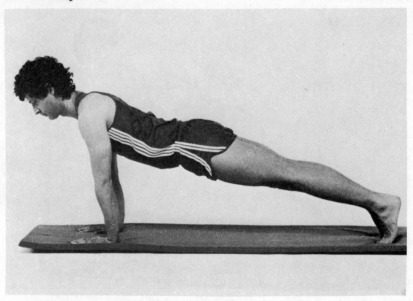

The universal exercise for building the arms: push-ups.

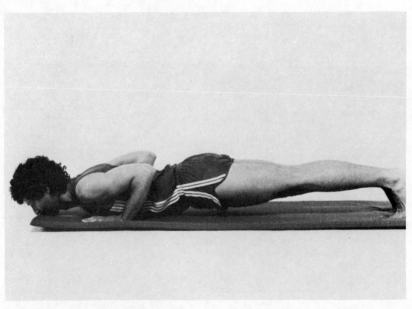

Keep your back straight, tail tucked.

19. Yoga Arm Balance

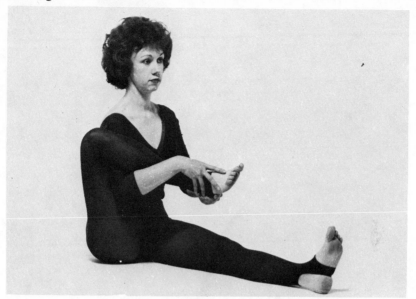

Yoga Arm Balance should be called Soft Pretzel.

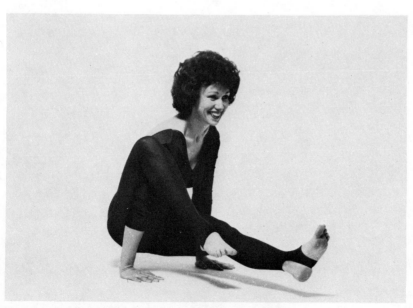

Your right arm is supposed to support your right leg, this way.

8

Cooldowns

"Don't stop, don't lie down, don't sit! Think about race horses; what do they do after they've run? Do they suddenly stop and sit down? Don't they have beautiful, strong legs?"

Even though I was only twelve years old when I heard those words from my gym class instructor, I haven't forgotten them, or their importance. My coach's bellowing insights marked my first awareness of the importance of cooling down after vigorous exercise. I had grown up near a race horse track, and so I had learned at an early age the proper treatment of a good race horse. By describing the training pattern of a thoroughbred race horse, the coach's instructions hit home.

Stretching and conditioning exercises are not just valuable for warming up then. There are exercises that allow the body to gradually slow down and relax. Actually, cooling down may be easier, initially, to incorporate into your training than warming up. After going for a run, your muscles have increased circulation and seem more receptive to stretching actions. The repeated contractions necessitated by the running action, however, have produced a tighter body than you had prior to your run. The back of the body is highly susceptible to tightening. Running also causes the major joints to compress and their surrounding ligaments to shorten. Stretching is important after running in order to regain the flexibility you had before the run. By forgoing exercises to cool you down, the muscular tension that results from running will continue. These tight, inflexible muscles make you more susceptible to injury and painful stiffening.

The exercises in this chapter are designed to help you recapture flexibility, but they also are useful in overcoming fatigue. Several of them call for elevating the legs or bringing the head down toward the feet (for improved venous drainage). Either position can help relieve the general feeling of languor, while reversing the effect that running has of pooling blood in the lower body.

Perhaps one of the most advantageous cool-down techniques is walking. Remember the race horse—your muscles are every bit as valuable as the winner of the Kentucky Derby.

COOLDOWNS

1. Pelvic Tilt

1. Lie on your back, knees bent, legs slightly apart, feet parallel. Place arms at side, palms down. Slide shoulder blades toward buttocks.

2. Exhale, contract buttocks, press lower back to floor. Hold for two breaths. Repeat several times.

Benefits: Relieves tension in lower back.

2. Downward Dog With Wall

1. Kneel by wall. Make a "V" with the thumb and fingers of each hand and place hands against wall, thumbs pointing toward each other. Hands are shoulder-width apart. Turn toes under.

2. Do Downward Dog (p.31). Press against wall and roll inner elbows under and out. When heels are down, lift toes for a few moments to intensify stretch. Hold fifteen to twenty seconds. Build to one minute.

3. Another way to use the wall in Downward Dog is to place your heels on the wall, toes on floor. Point fingers forward as in the regular Downward Dog.

Benefits: Using the wall enables you to work on straightening the arms or legs, giving a more intense stretch.

3. Big Toe Hanging Stretch

1. Stand in Growing Taller, feet slightly apart, and lift arms up.

2. Exhale and do Hanging Stretch (p.33) without holding the elbows. Straighten legs and raise kneecaps. Hold the big toes with the thumb and next two fingers of each hand, palms facing.

3. Exhale, bend elbows, bring chest to thighs, face to shins. Keep abdomen relaxed, legs straight. Hold for a few breaths, release. Come up as in Hanging Stretch.

Benefits: Stretches hamstrings and back.

4. Side Stretch I

1. Stand an arm's length from bench or chair. With hands on chair, place right foot in line between hands on floor. Step left foot back three feet directly in line with right foot. Turn left foot out thirty degrees.

2. Exhale, draw buttocks back, keeping hips even, legs straight. Arms are straight. Your weight should be evenly distributed though your feet. Keep moving right hip slightly back to align hips. Hold ten to fifteen seconds. Reverse.

Benefits: Good stretch for legs, arms, back. Increases awareness of movement in Side Stretch II.

5. Side Stretch II

1. Stand with feet parallel and 3 - 3½ feet apart. Bend elbows and hold wrists behind you. Tuck tail under, lift chest. Turn left foot in thirty degrees, right leg out ninety degrees. Turn upper body to face right leg.

2. Inhale, lift chest, roll shoulders back. Exhale, bend from the hips with a flat back. Keep legs straight. The weight should be evenly distributed through the feet, so press down on the ball of the front foot, heel on back. Draw the right hip back to align hips. Stop bending forward when you feel the back rounding (eventually the chest rests on the thigh). Hold for a few breaths. Reverse.

Benefits: Intense stretch for legs and hips. Improves posture.

6. Spread Leg Stretch I

1. Stand an arm's length from chair. Place the feet 4½ - 5 feet apart. Keep them parallel or turned slightly in.

2. Exhale, hold chair, straighten arms and back by lifting buttocks. Lift kneecaps to keep legs straight. Hold ten to fifteen seconds. Release.

Benefits: Stretches entire leg, strengthens ankles and feet. Prepares you for movement in Spread Leg Stretch II.

7. Spread Leg Stretch II

1. Stand with feet apart as in Spread Leg Stretch.

2. Exhale, place fingers on floor, palms toward you, hands in line with shoulders. (If possible, place hands between feet.)

3. Inhale, lift head, breastbone, and tailbone to concave, or flatten the back.

4. Exhale, keeping back flat, bend elbows, press down through the wrists, and bring head toward floor. Lower and upper arms should form right angles. Hold for a few breaths with straight legs. Release by straightening arms, place hands at the hips, and come up with a flat back.

Benefits: Stretches entire leg and back, strengthens ankles and feet.

1. Pelvic Tilt

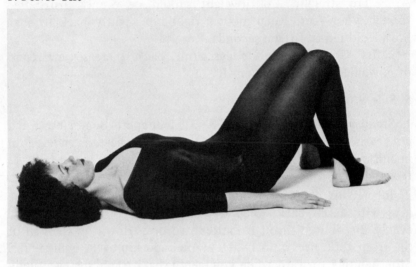

Pelvic Tilt relieves tension in lower back. Contract buttocks.

2. Downward Dog With Wall

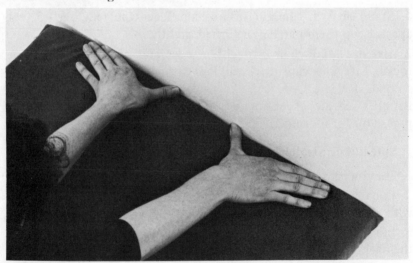

Place hands against a wall in Downward Dog With Wall.

2. Downward Dog With Wall (CONT'D.)

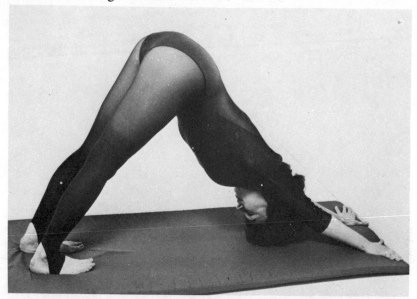

Assume Downward Dog position against wall.

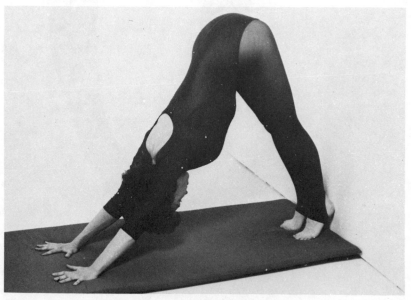

You can reverse position and place your heels against the wall.

3. Big Toe Hanging Stretch

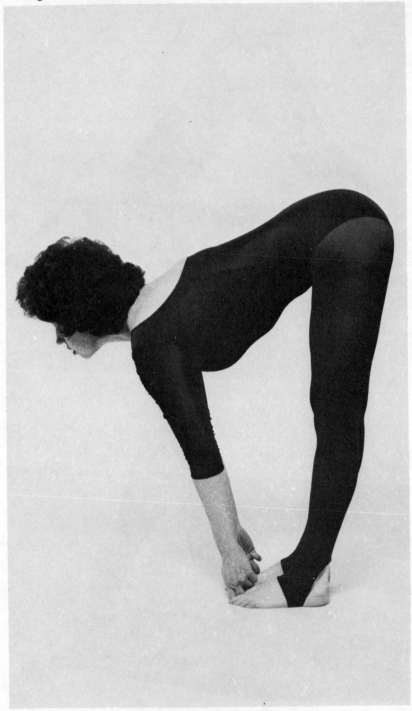

Place hands on floor and keep legs straight in Big Toe Hanging Stretch.

3. Big Toe Hanging Stretch (CONT'D.)

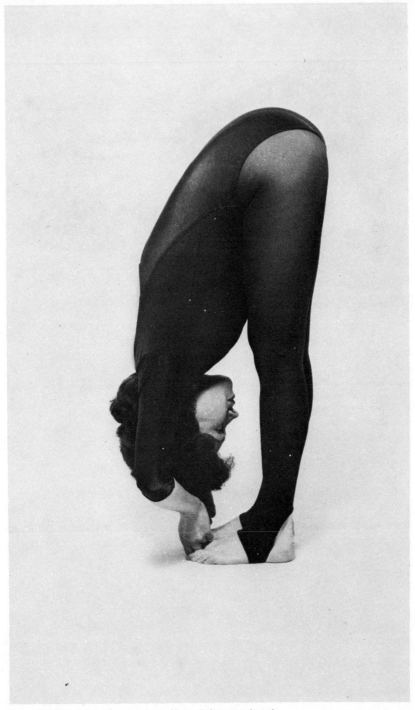

Bring chest to thighs, face to shins. Keep abdomen relaxed.

4. Side Stretch I

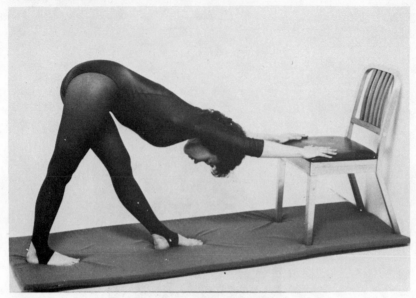

Bend at hips and place hands on a chair in Side Stretch I.

5. Side Stretch II

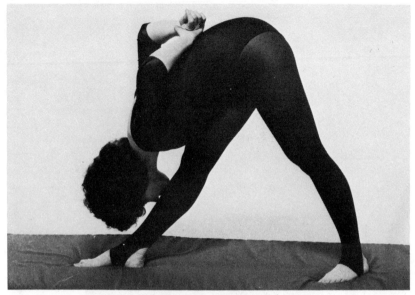

Side Stretch II improves posture. Touch your chest to your thigh.

6. Spread Leg Stretch I

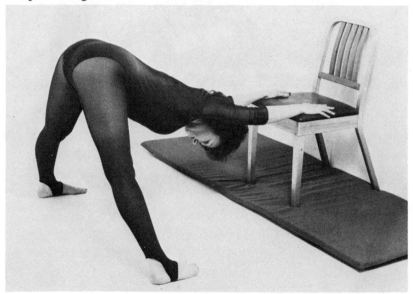

As you hold a chair, spread your legs wide for Spread Leg Stretch I.

7. Spread Leg Stretch II

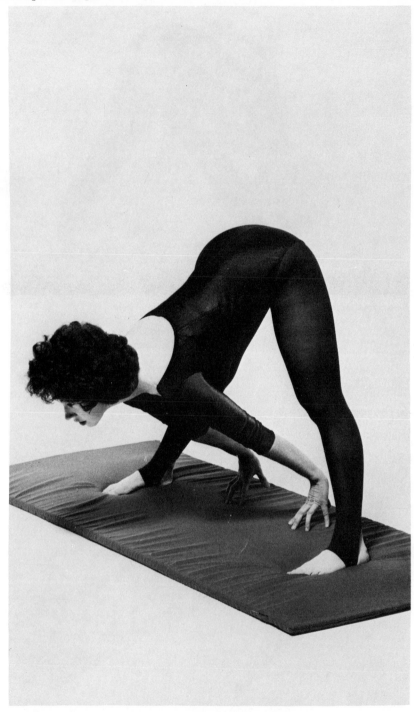

Spread legs and place fingers between legs to begin Spread Leg Stretch II.

7. Spread Leg Stretch II (CONT'D.)

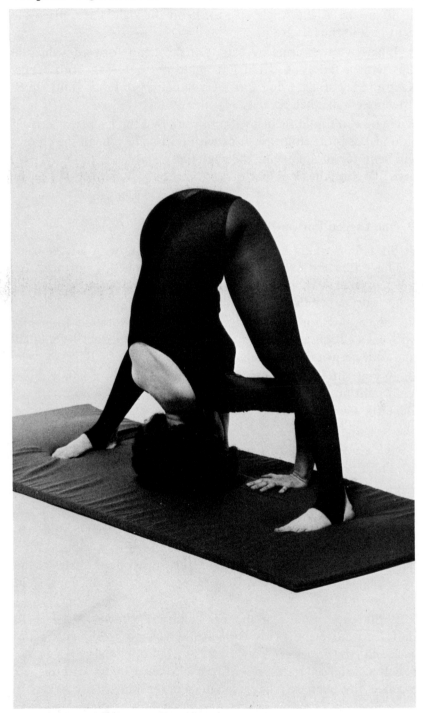

Bring head toward the floor and keep legs straight.

8. Half Forward Bend

1. Sit in the Right Angle (p. 87). Bend the right knee, place the right heel in the left groin.

2. Inhale, stretch arms by ears. Exhale, bend forward from the hips with a flat back. Hold left ankle or foot with both hands. Keep the leg straight and foot perpendicular to floor. Hold ten to fifteen seconds, then reverse.

3. If you can't hold the leg without rounding the back, use a towel around the foot. Hold the ends with both hands, bend the elbows and bend forward, keeping the back flat.

Benefits: Stretches legs, back.

9. One Legged Forward Bend

1. Sit as in Sitting Challenge V position (p. 61) with left leg back, right leg free and extended on floor. Left foot is by buttocks, left knee parallel with right knee. Balance equally on buttocks, keep right foot perpendicular with floor.

2. Inhale, lift arms along ears. Exhale, bend forward from hips with a flat back as in Half Forward Bend. Keep right leg straight and foot perpendicular. Hold ten to fifteen seconds. Reverse,

3. If you tilt to the right in this exercise, shove a pillow under your right buttock.

Benefits: Good stretch for feet, legs and back.

10. Full Forward Bend

1. Sit in Right Angle position. Keep the legs straight and the feet perpendicular to the floor during this exercise.

2. Inhale, stretch arms up by ears. Lift the chest and tip the pelvis forward. Exhale, bend forward from the hips, working with a flat back. Hold the big toes or place the fingers on the soles of the feet, fingers pointing down. Rest ribs on legs, face on shins. Hold for a few breaths.

3. If the back rounds or the legs bend, use a towel or belt as in Half Forward Bend. This will enable you to work with a flat back and straight legs.

Benefits: Intense stretch of entire backside of body. With regular practice, this exercise relieves fatigue and tension.

8. Half Forward Bend

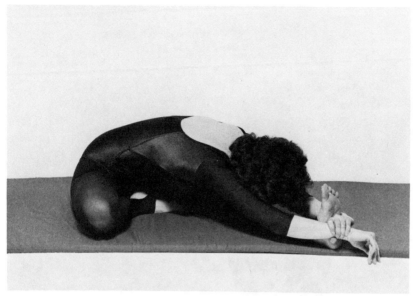

Tuck one leg in Half Forward Bend and then hold your straight leg at the ankle with your hands.

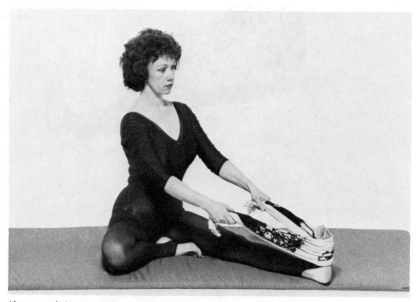

If you can't keep your back straight, use a towel around the foot.

9. One Legged Forward Bend

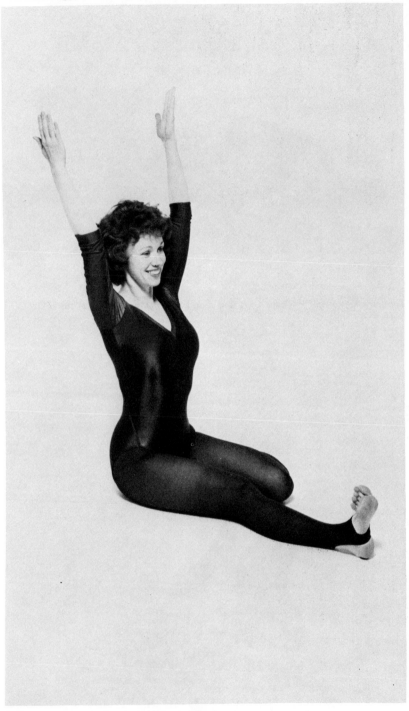

One leg is tucked in One Legged Forward Bend.

9. One Legged Forward Bend (CONT'D.)

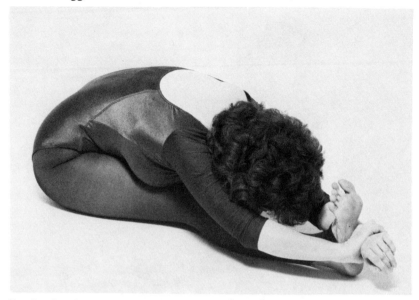

Now bend at the waist and bring your face toward the floor.

10. Full Forward Bend

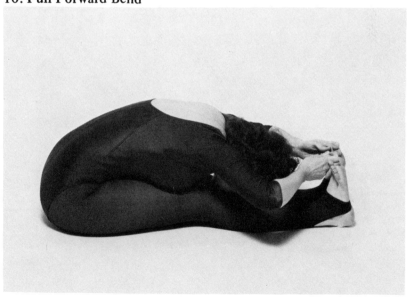

In Full Forward Bend, try to touch your nose to the floor.

(CONT'D NEXT PAGE)

10. Full Forward Bend (CONT'D.)

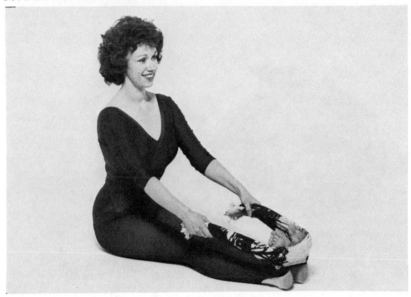

If the back rounds in Full Forward Bend, use a towel.

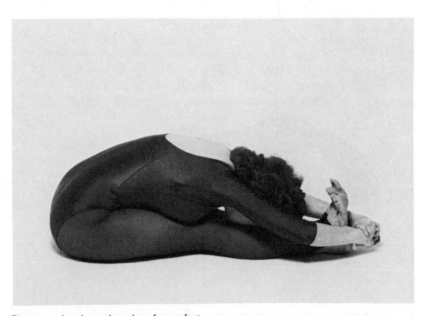

Place your hands on the soles of your feet.

11. Wide Angle Forward Bend I.

1. Sit in position of Right Angle (p. 87). Spread legs wide apart. Keep the legs straight, the feet vertical. Tilt the pelvis forward.

2. Inhale, stretch the arms up along ears. Exhale, bend forward from the hips with a flat back. Take a few breaths.

3. Exhale, hold the ankles or big toes. Take a few breaths, then release. (This stretch may also be done with the arms staying by the ears, palms on the floor.)

Benefits: Intense stretch for the back and legs.

12. Wide Angle Forward Bend II

1. Sit in Right Angle position. Spread legs wide apart as in Wide Angle Forward Bend I.

2. Inhale, lift arms up and turn torso to face right leg.

3. Exhale, bend forward from the hips with a flat back. Hold the right foot with both hands. Both legs remain straight, weight stays on both buttocks. Take a few breaths, then release. Reverse.

Benefits: Excellent stretch for back, hips and inner legs.

13. Standing Splits

1. Do Downward Dog.

2. Exhale, keep right leg straight and lift it as high as possible. Right knee faces floor, right buttock level with left. Hold for a few breaths, then release. Reverse.

Benefits: Stretches hamstrings, Achilles tendon, calf muscles. Arms and shoulders are stretched and strengthened.

14. Wall Standing Split

1. Do Downward Dog with heels against the wall.

2. Exhale, lift the right leg and place right knee and foot on wall. Rest of body in Downward Dog. Take a few breaths. If this is easy go to step 3. If step 2 is a good stretch for you, change legs.

3. Exhale, straighten right leg with toes turned under on wall. Keep buttocks level. Hold for a few breaths. Release and change sides.

Benefits: Intense stretch for leg and groin.

11. Wide Angle Forward Bend I

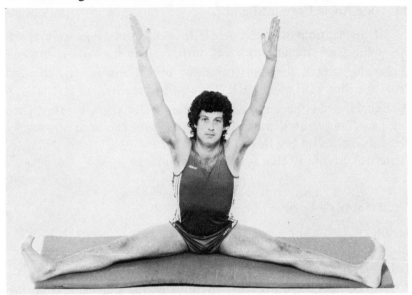

Sit in position of Right Angle, for Wide Angle Forward Bend I, and hold the ankles with your hands. Bend at the waist.

12. Wide Angle Forward Bend II

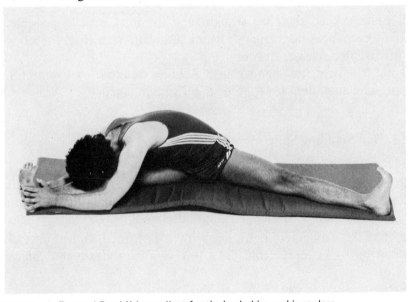

Wide Angle Forward Bend II is excellent for the back, hips and inner legs.

13. Standing Splits

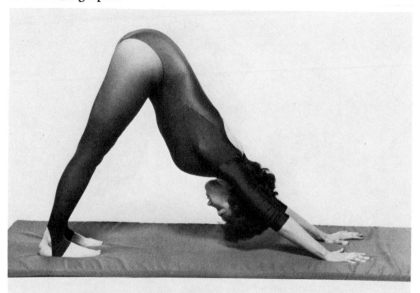

To begin Standing Splits start with Downward Dog.

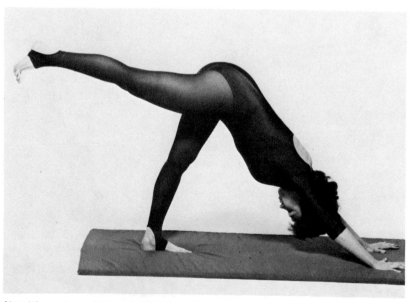

Now lift one leg as high as possible; keep it straight.

14. Wall Standing Split

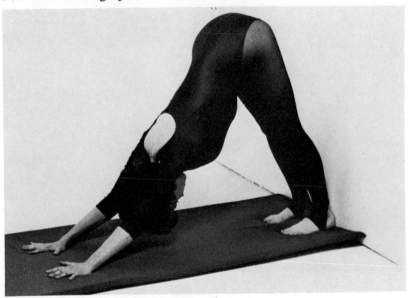

Wall Standing Split is an intense stretch for the leg and groin.

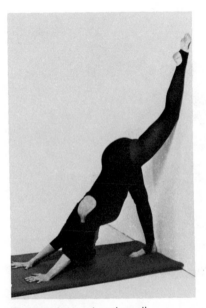

Place one foot against the wall.

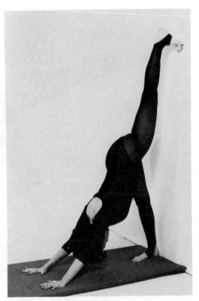

Now straighten your leg, raising the foot up against the wall.

15. Reverse Triangle

1. Stand with feet 3 - 3½ feet apart. Turn left foot in sixty degrees, right leg out ninety degrees. Align feet as in Triangle (p. 20). Stretch arms out horizontally.

2. Exhale, swing the left side around to the right. Bend from the hips and place the left fingertips on the floor beside the right foot. Fingers point parallel with the foot. With both legs straight, press down on the back heel and ball of the front foot. Expand the chest, stretch the right shoulder and right arm up, left shoulder and left arm down, to form a vertical line. Extend the back horizontally. Hold for a few breaths. Swing up and reverse.

3. If you can't touch the floor with straight legs, place a book or a chair under the hand.

Benefits: Strengthens and stretches the legs. Loosens the hips and releases lower-back tension.

16. Knee Twists

1. Lie on your back with arms in a "T" position. Bend your knees to your chest to flatten the lower back.

2. Exhale, roll the knees to the right, inhale up, and then exhale them to the left. Keep shoulders down. Repeat five to ten times.

Benefits: Releases lower-back tension.

17. Wall Shoulder Stand

1. Lie on your side on a padded surface with buttocks touching the wall, knees bent. Roll over to your back, stretch legs up wall. Place your feet on the wall. Feet slightly apart and parallel. Place arms along body, palms down.

2. Exhale, press down on the arms and lift buttocks up. Interlock your fingers and stretch hands toward wall. Keep feet flat on wall, knees in line with feet. Hold for a few breaths, then roll down. Do not turn your head during this exercise. If there is any strain on your neck, try placing your head off the mat as in Shoulder Stand.

Benefits: Loosens shoulders; good preparation for inverting the body in Shoulder Stand.

15. Reverse Triangle

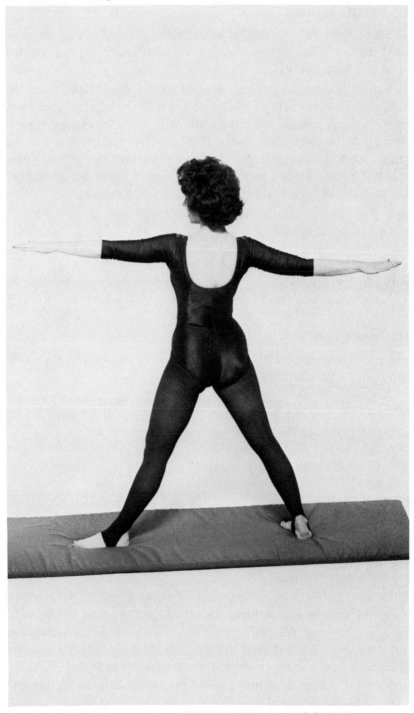

Reverse Triangle is a more complex version of one often done in P.E. classes.

15. Reverse Triangle (CONT'D.)

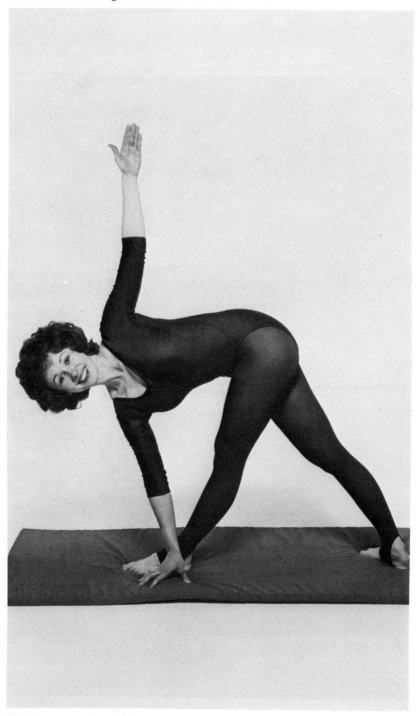

This gives tremendous stretch to the torso and legs.

15. Reverse Triangle (CONT'D.)

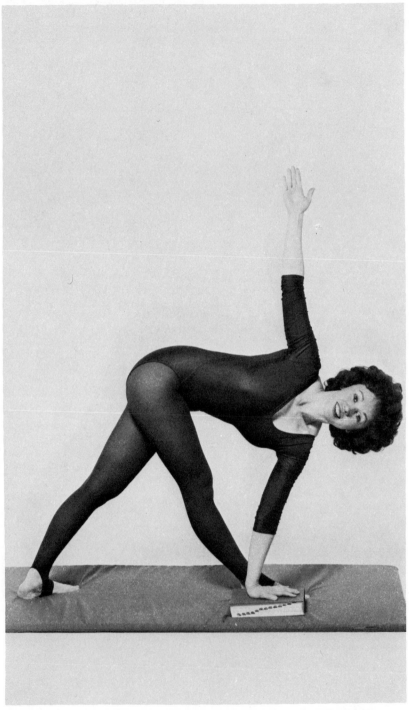

Swing up and reverse position. Place a book under the hand if you can't reach the floor.

16. Knee Twists

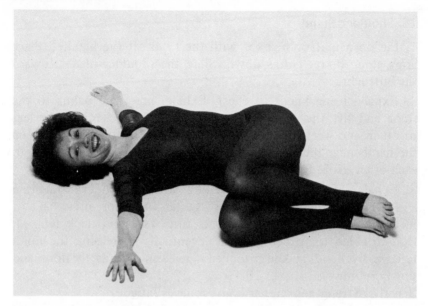

Knee Twists releases lower-back tension.

17. Wall Shoulder Stand

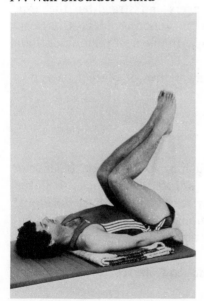

Wall Shoulder Stand puts strain on the neck, so be careful.

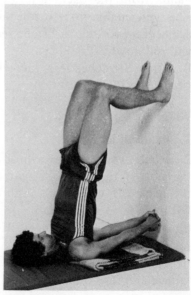

Keep feet flat on the wall. Loosens shoulders.

18. Shoulder Stand

1. Lie on a mat or blanket with the head off the blanket. Place arms along body, palms down. Slide the shoulder blades toward the buttocks.

2. Exhale, bring knees to chest. Exhale, press the palms to the floor and lift the hips, roll knees to forehead, keep lower legs together and vertical. Support the back with your hands. Keep the hands near the floor, fingers pointing up, little fingers close to each other. Hold for a few breaths.

3. Exhale, lift knees toward ceiling, tuck tail under, straighten legs. Keep legs and feet together, tighten kneecaps, press balls of feet toward ceiling. Keep buttocks firm, face and neck relaxed. Hold for ten to fifteen seconds, eventually increasing the hold. Release by bending knees to head, releasing hands to floor and slowly rolling down.

Benefits: Strengthens upper body, relieves fatigue.

19. Plough With Chair

1. Do the Shoulder Stand with a chair behind your head.

2. Exhale, bend the legs back over your face, balancing the tips of the toes on the chair. Place feet and legs together. Keep the legs straight and lift the buttocks to straighten the back. Release the hands from the back, interlock fingers and straighten the arms. This will enable you to roll higher on your shoulders. Hold back again. Hold for ten to fifteen seconds. Inhale up to Shoulder Stand and roll down.

Benefits: Stretches legs, increases awareness of correct back position in the Plough.

20. Plough

1. Do Shoulder Stand.

2. Exhale, bend legs over head, touching toes to floor. Balance on the tips of the toes. Straighten legs. Lift the buttocks to flatten the back. (If your back rounds or legs bend, go back to Plough With Chair (p.168). Keep a maximum distance between face and thighs. Relax face and neck. Hold ten to fifteen seconds, building to one minute.

Benefits: Stretches legs, strengthens and stretches spine, relieves fatigue and tension.

18. Shoulder Stand

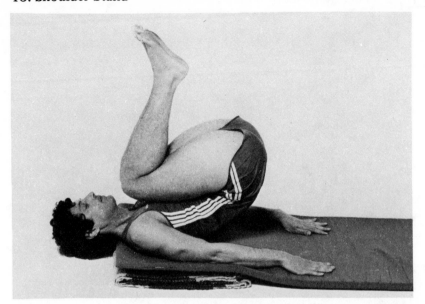

Lie on a mat to do Shoulder Stand, head off the mat.

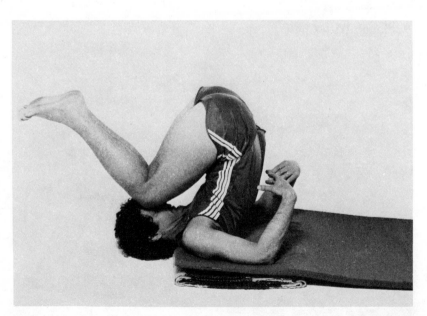

Bring your knees over your face as you start the movement.

(CONT'D NEXT PAGE)

18. Shoulder Stand (CONT'D.)

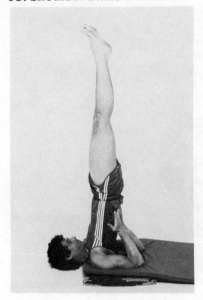

Now lift your legs to the sky and support your back with your hands.

19. Plough With Chair

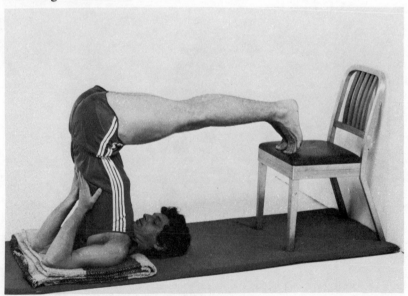

Do the Shoulder Stand to begin Plough With Chair.

19. Plough With Chair (CONT'D.)

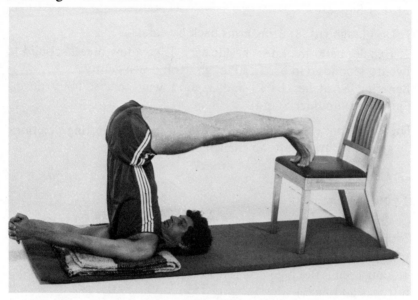

Release your hands from your back and put them on the mat.

20. Plough

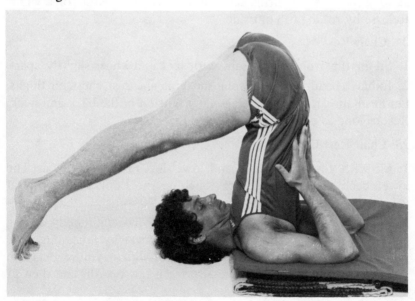

Try to keep legs straight when in Plough position.

21. Ear Squeeze

1. Do Plough (p.168) Bring arms back by ears.
2. Exhale, bend the knees beside ears. Take a few breaths; build to twenty seconds. Go back to Plough. Roll down gently.
Benefits: Stretches back, and a good way to rest body during Plough or Shoulder Stand.

The following exercises are very gentle and easy resting positions for relieving fatigue after a challenging workout.

22. Child's Rest

If your legs are flexible:

1. Kneel and rest your chest on your knees, head and arms on floor.
2. Exhale, relax the back, neck and face. Relax as long as you like. (If you aren't flexible, try the exercise with a pillow under the buttocks and face.)

23. Lazy Leg Stretch

1. Lie on your side, knees bent, buttocks near the wall.
2. Exhale, roll on your back, extend legs up wall. Keep the feet flat, arms away from body, palms up. Flatten the lower back.
3. Exhale, spread legs apart by sliding them down the wall. Stay as long as possible. Bring legs back to vertical. Rest for a while. Release by rolling to your side.

24. Chair Rest

1. Sit in the front of a chair, with feet and knees slightly apart.
2. Exhale, bend forward from the hips and rest chest on thighs. Let head and arms hang. Release any tension in the back and neck. Rest as long as possible.

25. Chair Rest On Back

1. Lie with your knees bent and lower legs resting on a chair. The lower back should be near or touching the floor. Place arms at your side, palms up. Close your eyes.
2. Exhale, relax your back, face and neck. Relax completely, letting go of any tension. Allow the body to recover by imagining your fatigue melting downward into the floor. When you're ready to sit up, roll over to your side, pause for a few breaths and then sit up.

21. Ear Squeeze

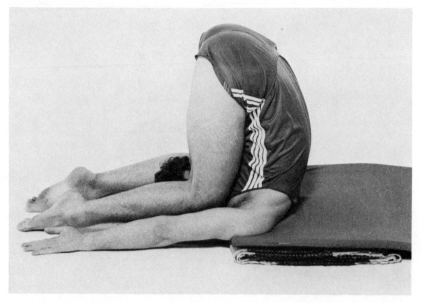

Ear Squeeze is an advanced form of the Plough.

22. Child's Rest

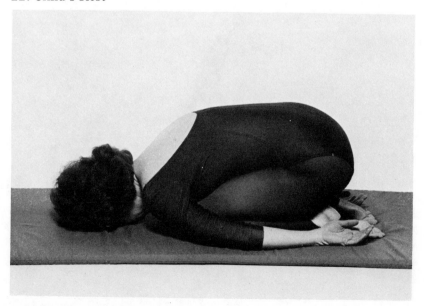

In Child's Rest, your chest should touch your knees.

23. Lazy Leg Stretch

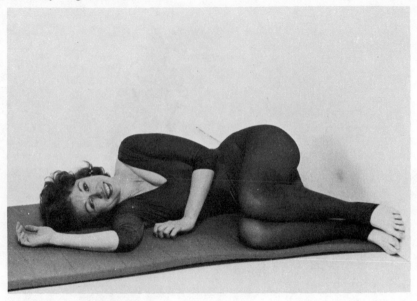

Lie on your side, legs bent, to begin Lazy Leg Stretch.

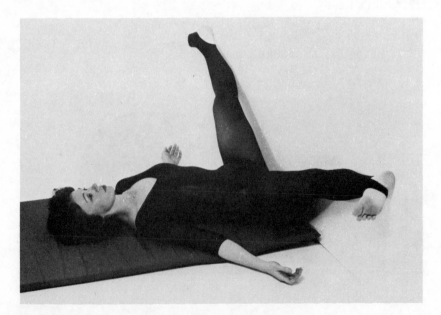

Roll on your back and extend legs up a wall. Spread legs.

24. Chair Rest

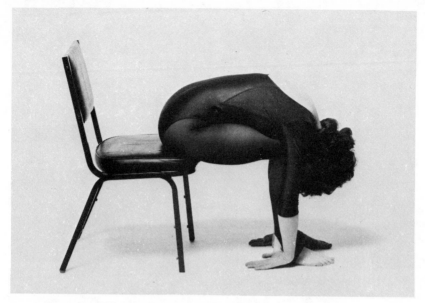

People who've had a hard day might try the Chair Rest.

25. Chair Rest On Back

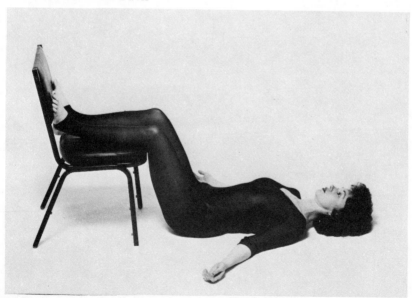

Chair Rest On Back is great for draining the legs of waste products after a hard run.

9

Six-Day Stretching and Conditioning Plan for the Runner

The following six-day exercise plan is a good way to start combining stretching and running. After a few weeks, you may want to adjust it to emphasize a particularly stiff or weak spot in your body. In fact, this plan should serve only as a guide. With regular stretching, you'll locate your problem areas. Focus on them by selecting exercises designed for those particular inflexibilities or weaknesses.

DAY 1

Growing Taller
Side Stretch
Back Extender
Leg Stretch
Rock N Roll
Ledge Stretch
Wall Chair
Squat Challenge I - III
Chorus Line

Walk—Run—Walk
Side Stretch I or II
Downward Dog With Wall
Big Toe Hanging Stretch
Camel
Wall Shoulder Stand
Right Angle
Half Forward Bend
Wide Angle Forward Bend
Wall Twist or Yoga Twist
Child's Rest

DAY 2

Kneeling Back Extender
Twisting Leg Stretch
Straight Leg Calf Stretch
Triangle
Groin Stretch
Growing Longer
Toe-Heel Stretch
Leg Lift I - III
Belly Twister I - II
Soft Pretzel
Walk—Run—Walk
Pelvic Tilts
Rock A Baby I or II
Indian Cobbler I or II
Downward Dog
Standing Splits
Standing Splits With Wall
Reverse Triangle
Splits
Shoulder Stand
Chair Rest On Back

DAY 3

Growing Taller
Arm Rotations
Invisible Chair
Bent Knee Calf Stretch
Chest Expander I - II
Cross Leg Rock N Roll
Hip Opener
Beginning Lateral Stretch or Extended Lateral Stretch
Closed Gate
Wall Hang
Roll Down Hang
Walk—Run—Walk
Spread Leg Stretch I - II
Downward Dog With Wall
One Arm Balance
Roll Ups
Hands Up Your Back
Bridge
Shoulder Stand
Plough With Chair
Chair Rest

DAY 4

Side Stretch
Back Extender
Wall Chest Opener
Straight Leg Calf Stretch
Runner's Stretch
Proud Warrior
Archer
Sitting Challenge I - V
Chorus Line
Walk—Run—Walk

Knee Twists
Resting Leg Stretch
Resting Leg Lift I - II
Supported Runner's Balance/Runner's Balance
Elbow-Arm Chest Stretch
Intense Front Stretch I or II
Shoulder Stand
Plough
Chair Rest On Back

DAY 5

Growing Taller
Dancer's Stretch I - IV
Rock N Roll
Boat Butterfly
Flat Boat
Heel In Toe Twist
Roll Down Hang
New Leg Balance
Walk—Run—Walk
Triangle
Thigh Stretch
Sitting Side Stretch
Beginning Lateral Stretch or Extended Lateral Stretch
Reverse Triangle
Wall Shoulder Stand
One Legged Forward Bend
Full Forward Bend

DAY 6

Yoga Warm-Up (three to six cycles)
Prone Back Leg Lift
Prone Body Lift
Bow
Standing Bow
Walk–Run–Walk
Downward Dog
Push-Ups (any type)
Tree
Backward Groin Stretch
High Bridge
Plough With Chair
Wide Angle Forward Bend I - II
Chair Twist I or II
Chair Rest On Back

10

Core Programs for Other Sports

The core programs are exercise sequences to enhance and improve your enjoyment of your sport. The program may be used before or after your sports activity. Try it for a week, and then begin substituting other exercises as you adjust the program to your body's needs.

BACKPACKING

Leg Stretch
Ledge Stretch
Toe-Heel Stretch
Yoga Warm Up (3 - 6 cycles)
Triangle
Proud Warrior
Wall/Invisible Chair
Push-Ups
Squat Challenge I - III
Boat
Bridge

Camel
Shoulder Stand
Plough
Forward Bend (any)

BASEBALL

Yoga Warm-Up (3 - 6 cycles)
The Dancer
Wall Chest Opener
Hands On Your Back
Intense Front Stretch I - II
One Arm Balance
Push-Ups
Archer
Squat Challenge I - III
Dancer's Stretch I - IV
Standing Bow
Supported Runner's Balance
Tree

BICYCLING

Back Extender
Bent Knee/Straight Leg Calf Stretch
Leg Stretch
Triangle
Wall/Invisible Chair
The Dancer
Sitting Challenge I - IV
Standing Bow
Prone Body Lift
Bow
Downward Dog
Push-Ups
Shoulder Stand
Plough

Half Forward Bend
One Legged Forward Bend
Full Forward Bend

BOATING

Back Extender
Elbow-Arm Chest Stretch
Chest Expander I - II
Yoga Warm-Up (3 - 6 cycles)
Triangle
Extended Lateral Stretch
Reverse Triangle
Prone Body Lift
Bridge
Camel
Boat
Chair Twists

BOWLING

Growing Taller
Side Stretch
Downward Dog
Toe-Heel Stretch
Groin Stretch
Arm Rotations
Elbow-Arm Chest Stretch
Blanket Roll
Table Hang
Pelvic Tilt
Bridge
Spread Leg Stretch
Wide Angle Forward Bend
Chair Twists

DOWNHILL SKIING

Bent Knee/Straight Leg Calf Stretch
Dancer's Stretch I - IV
Wall/Invisible Chair
Triangle
Extended Lateral Stretch
Proud Warrior
The Dancer
Squat Challenge I - III
Sitting Challenge I - V
Prone Body Lift
Backward Groin Stretch
Bow
Bridge
Hip Opener
Archer
Downward Dog
Push-Ups
Leg Lifts
Boat
Forward Bend (any)
Intense Hanging Stretch
Wall/Standing Splits
Chorus Line
Wall/Yoga Twist

GOLF

Growing Taller
Leg Stretch
Dancer's Stretch I - IV
Toe-Heel Stretch
Roll-Ups
Rock N Roll
Leg Lifts

Pelvic Tilt
Bridge
Yoga Warm-Up (2 - 4 cycles)
Triangle
Elbow-Arm Chest Stretch
Chest Expander I - II
Hands On Your Back
Knee Twists
Chair Twists
Wall Twist

HORSEBACK RIDING

Side Stretch
Dancer's Stretch I - IV
Triangle
Proud Warrior
Groin Stretch
Sitting Challenge I - V
Resting Leg Lift I - II
Archer
Downward Dog
Boat
Indian Cobbler I - II
Hip Opener
Closed Gate
Tree
Runner's Balance
New Leg Balance

RACKET SPORTS

Arm Rotations
Back Extender
Elbow-Arm Chest Stretch
Hands On Your Back

The Dancer
Triangle
Proud Warrior
Wall/Invisible Chair
Squat Challenge I - III
Hip Opener
Archer

SKATING

Ledge Stretch
Yoga Warm-Up (4 - 8 cycles)
Push-Ups
Triangle
Extended Lateral Stretch
Proud Warrior
Runner's Balance
New Leg Balance
Tree
Sitting Challenge I - V
Squat Challenge I - III
Bridge
Camel
Shoulder Stand
Plough
Standing Splits
Wide Angle Forward Bend I - II

SWIMMING

Back Extender
Downward Dog
Ledge Stretch
Triangle
Extended Lateral Stretch
New Leg Balance

Roll Down Hang
Prone Back Leg Lift
Prone Body Lift
Bow
Standing Bow
Hands On Your Back
Squat Challenge I - III
Intense Front Stretch
Bridge
Push-Ups
Boat
Half Forward Bend
Full Forward Bend
Chair Twists

WATER SKIING

Back Extender
Ledge Stretch
Toe-Heel Stretch
Yoga Warm-Up (3 - 6 cycles)
Triangle
Proud Warrior
Wall Chair
Elbow-Arm Chest Stretch
Squat Challenge I - III
Push-Ups
Roll-Ups
Leg Lifts
Hands On Your Back
Prone Body Lift
Bridge
Camel
One Arm Balance
Spread Leg Stretch I - II

WEIGHTLIFTING

Hands On your Back
Archer
Rock N Roll
Dancer's Stretch I - IV
Runner's Balance
Triangle
Extended Lateral Stretch
Side Stretch I - II
Yoga Warm-Up (2 - 4 cycles)
Sitting Challenge I - V
Camel
Hip Opener
Closed Gate
Prone Body Lift
Shoulder Stand
Plough
Spread Leg Stretch
Forward Bend (any)
Wall Twist

About the Author

Nell Weaver is a free-lance writer and yoga teacher. She is the co-author of *Runner's World Yoga Book*. Nell has an M.A. in English and Communications, and has worked in television public relations and as a college teacher.

A veteran hiker, she has taken many backpacking and cross-country ski trips in the Pacific Northwest and Alaska. She lived in Great Britain for two years, has visited India and the Soviet Union, and has hiked and traveled extensively throughout Europe.

Nell lives in Little Rock, Arkansas, with her husband, Bob, their Airedale, Phoebe, and an Alaskan house cat, Peter.

Recommended Reading

ALEXANDER TECHNIQUE, by Wilfred Barlow. Alfred A. Knopf, Inc., New York, NY, 1973. A technique that teaches body realignment. Habitual, incorrect posture and harmful movements are discussed.

AWARENESS THROUGH MOVEMENT, by Moshe Feldenkrais. Harper and Row, New York, NY, 1977. Method incorporating simple exercises to improve body alignment and increase self-awareness.

DOUBLE YOGA: A NEW SYSTEM FOR TOTAL BODY HEALTH, by Ganga White with Anna Forrest. Penguin Books, New York, NY, 1981. A good book for experienced yoga students who want to work with a partner. Beautifully illustrated.

THE FOOT BOOK, by Harry F. Hlavac. World Publications, Mountain View, CA, 1977. A one-volume encyclopedia of the foot. Valuable reference guide containing technical information and practical advice.

HOW TO DOCTOR YOUR FEET WITHOUT THE DOCTOR, by Myles J. Schneider and Mark Sussman. Charles Scribner's Sons, New York, NY, 1980. Well-illustrated guide that discusses the role of flexibility in maintaining healthy feet, knees, hips and back. Highly recommended for runners and walkers.

JANE FONDA'S WORKOUT BOOK, by Jane Fonda. Simon and Schuster, New York, NY, 1981. A woman's personal celebration of the joys of being strong, healthy and fit. Exercises are set to music.

LIGHT ON YOGA, by B.K.S. Iyengar. Schocken Books, New York, NY, 1966 (Revised edition, 1977). The classic, definitive guide to yoga. Over six hundred illustrations. Iyengar's instructions, hints, and cautions are based on the experiences of more than forty years of teaching.

LILIAS, YOGA, AND YOUR LIFE, by Lilias Folan. Macmillan Publishing Co., Inc., New York, NY, 1981. A clear, easy-to-use guide.

NEW EXERCISES FOR RUNNERS, by the editors of *Runner's World*, World Publications, Mountain View, CA, 1978. A succinct, practical book with chapters on stretching.

RUNNER'S WORLD INDOOR EXERCISE BOOK, by Rich Benyo and Rhonda Provost. World Publications, Mountain View, CA, 1981. A beginner's guide to fitness.

RUNNER'S WORLD YOGA BOOK, by Jean Couch with Nell Weaver. World Publications, Mountain View, CA, 1979. The yogic approach to exercise and health. Originally conceived as an introductory text for athletes, this book has also become popular with yoga enthusiasts.

ROLFING, by Ida Rolf. Dennis-Landman, Santa Monica, CA, 1977. Rolf's analysis of the desirable healthy body's alignment.

STRETCHING, by Bob Anderson. Shelter Publications, Bolinas, CA, 1980. A comprehensive look at stretching that includes helpful drawings and programs for specific sports.